The Soul's Palette

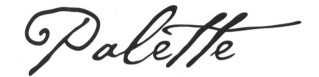

The Soul's Palette

DRAWING ON ART'S TRANSFORMATIVE POWERS FOR HEALTH AND WELL-BEING

Cathy A. Malchiodi

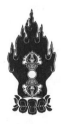

SHAMBHALA

BOSTON & LONDON

2002

Shambhala Publications, Inc.
Horticultural Hall
300 Massachusetts Avenue
Boston, Massachusetts 02115
www.shambhala.com

9 8 7 6 5 4

Printed in the United States of America

∞ This edition is printed on acid-free paper that meets the American
National Standards Institute Z39.48 Standard.

♻ This book was printed on 30% postconsumer recycled paper.
For more information please visit us at www.shambhala.com.

Distributed in the United States by Random House, Inc., and in
Canada by Random House of Canada Ltd

Interior design and composition: Greta D. Sibley & Associates

Library of Congress Cataloging-in-Publication Data
Malchiodi, Cathy A.
The soul's palette: drawing on art's transformative powers for health
and well-being / Cathy A. Malchiodi.
p. cm.
Includes bibliographical references.
ISBN 978-1-57062-815-3 (pbk.)
1. Arts—Therapeutic use. I. Title.
RM931.A77 M35 2002
615.8'5156—dc21
2002003895

For my mother, Grace Malchiodi,
who introduced me to the wonder and miracle
of crayons, paper, and paints.

Contents

Preface

During the time I was writing this book, terror gripped America while a nation hypnotically watched broadcasts of planes crashing into the World Trade Center in New York City, the Pentagon in Washington, D.C., and a field in rural Pennsylvania. Images of terrorist attacks, collapsing buildings, and fireballs repeated themselves hundreds of times on the instant replay of television, imprinting our hearts with fear and shocking the depths of our senses. The pictures of survivors, firefighters, police, doctors, and nurses that followed stirred our compassion and brought us together to mourn those who died in the days following the tragedy.

Traumatized by the horror of what I saw and felt, I went to my studio to try to make sense of my experiences. With profound sadness I painted the gray smoke and ashes I witnessed on September 11, 2001, thinking of the thousands of souls who died on that day. A few days later, I painted a frightening and chaotic image of a recurring nightmare I had about bloodshed, mass devastation, and my own death in a nuclear war. Soon after, I returned to my studio to paint an image of an angel after hearing a man tell me how he lost his entire family at the World Trade Center collapse. Two months after the terrorist attacks, I painted a large, luminous globe of clear light surrounded by gold, an image that gave me a sense of peace and safety. As I now look back on these paintings, I find myself once again humbled by the power of image making and imagination. I literally painted my way out my despair, fear, and mourning, and reexperienced the miracle that artistic creativity has to heal and transform during the darkest hours of the soul.

In the days that followed September 11, others, too, experienced this miracle, and art and symbols appeared, spontaneously emerging as a therapy for the very images that traumatized so many. Union Square, a well-known landmark in New York City, became a living museum of imagery in tribute to the victims of the attacks. A student brought mural paper that was soon covered with images and prayers. Two Armenian immigrants arrived with an eight-foot column they had created as a memorial; photos of the missing and candles, flowers, and cards immediately surrounded its base. In response to the terrifying pictures of destruction and death witnessed only two days before, people used symbols and images to express sorrow, support, and hope.

Art's true function is to inspire us, mirror our thoughts, and embody our emotions. When words are not enough, we turn to image and symbol to speak for us. They are a conduit to all we contain within and a way of reflecting and recounting where we have been, where we are, and where we are going. Artistic expression is far more than self-expression and has much more astonishing power. Artistic creativity offers a source of inner wisdom that can provide guidance, soothe emotional pain, and revitalize your being. More important, it is a wellspring that enlivens, rejuvenates, restores, and transforms and it exists within everyone for health and well-being. Expressing yourself in deceptively simple ways—through drawings, paintings, sculptures, photography—uncovers this natural medicine within. By tapping your creative source, your ability to express yourself through images, you come to know yourself more fully and deeply, access the intuitive powers within you to heal, and naturally nurture the soul. Quite simply, art is good for you and may be as important to your overall health as balanced nutrition, regular exercise, or meditation.

Since ancient times, art has served as a means to repair and renew the self, and the world's wisdom traditions have affirmed imagery as a remedy for what ails body and mind. While images have always been used to restore well-being, the power of the creative imagination is only now being recognized as an integral healing agent. It is being embraced within the equation of wellness and health maintenance and is experiencing a rebirth in hospitals, clinics, and rehabilitation centers. Healing art, art therapy, arts medicine, and arts in health care are some of the names coined to describe our rapidly growing understanding of how images and image making can guide, transform, and heal. As medicine embraces more integrative forms of treatment, we are recognizing that creative expression is a long-standing and fundamental source of health and wellness for body, emotions, mind, and spirit.

For some twenty years I have witnessed the healing power of art in people of all ages. Whether it is an abused child intuitively scribbling the horror of her trauma on paper, a group of breast cancer survivors painting rage and fear, or a father overcome with the death of his child creating memorial sculpture in his backyard, all have encountered the transformative capacity of art and image. Each has tapped the ancient wisdom of image and imagination. All have discovered that art helps us to make meaning in powerful and dramatic ways, conveys our deepest feelings, gives voice to our spirit, and helps us to transcend suffering and touch something beyond ourselves. They have reconnected with the soul's palette, the creative source within that heals, makes whole, and helps us deeply understand who we are in a way that no other way of knowing can.

My personal journey to understand why art and imagination heal has led me to explore and develop creative and easily accessible activities that anyone can use. They are inspired by spiritual practices, influenced by wellness paradigms, and based on a belief that creativity is a healing force. While I encourage you to try as many of these activities as possible, let your intuition and curiosity be your guide to what feels right for you as you read this book. And know that you already have within you everything you need to fully experience the miracle of your artistic creativity as a source of wisdom, transformation, and well-being.

Acknowledgments

Writing a book is not a solitary journey but one that is guided and shaped by family, good friends, colleagues, and mentors along the way. The following individuals made writing this book possible through their support and wisdom:

My mother, Grace, for nurturing my soul's palette, and my father, James, for giving me the opportunity to explore and pursue a career in art.

My husband, David, for his love and support, without which I could not have found the time or the energy to pursue my dream of being an author.

Friend, colleague, and fellow writer Shaun McNiff, for reading the manuscript at its tender, unedited stage and for cheering me on with generosity, praise, and humor.

Individuals whose wisdom and friendship have made my life richer and encouraged my work as a therapist, artist, and author, and challenged my thinking: Shirley Riley, Susan Spaniol, Frances Kaplan, Lori Vance, Pat Allen, Michael Franklin, Holly Feen-Calligan, Bill

Steele, Carol Thayer Cox, Anna Riley-Hiscox, Linney Wix, Rochelle Serwator, and Jessica Kingsley.

The children, adults, and families in my art therapy practice who have shown me on countless occasions the powers of art and the creative process to repair, restore, and transform.

I extend thanks to the following individuals for giving permission to use their illustrations throughout this book: Annette Reynolds, Deborah Koff-Chapin, Shirley Riley, Don Lambert, Pria Campanelli, Kit Jenkins and Mary Flannery of RAW Artworks, Kendra Crossen Burroughs, and Allison and Alex Grey. Thank you, Ewa Wasilewska, for last-minute photography and unwavering support of my work.

Finally, I want to express special gratitude to Kendra Crossen Burroughs, whose editorial talents have shaped this book with the utmost professionalism, intelligence, and insight. I feel very fortunate to have had the opportunity to work with Kendra, who brought clarity to my thoughts and transformed them into beautifully constructed sentences when words failed me. If that were not enough, Kendra has a magnificent breadth of knowledge of art, psychology, and spiritual practices that contributed to the accuracy of each page of this work and challenged me to be more precise in my thinking and writing. Thank you, Kendra, and thank you, Shambhala Publications, both for giving me the chance to work with her and for believing in this book.

The Soul's Palette

ONE

Rediscovering the Soul's Palette

ART AND SOUL

When I was young, I learned through Catholicism that my soul was as important as my mind and body. I remember being instructed at weekly catechism to guard my immortal soul at all cost, and I sometimes worried that my soul might end up in the less desirable resting places of purgatory or hell rather than the celestial kingdom of heaven. To ensure my soul's admittance to heaven in the afterlife, my parents took me to weekly confession at the local church. There, any misdeeds or transgressions that could damage one's soul were told to the priest in preparation for receiving the sacrament of Holy Communion the next day. In the concrete mind of a child, I was in awe of our local priest's apparent power to absolve my soul of any sin and to magically cleanse that invisible entity inside me. After confession I would look in my bedroom mirror, narrow my eyes, and imagine that the aura I saw around my body was my purified soul leaking out around the edges.

I actually didn't know any other definitions of soul until I was a teenager. At Friday night school dances in junior high, one of my friends would do a fabulous impression of Soul Brother Number One, James Brown. I had never heard soul music before, but I knew immediately that its rhythms made me feel alive and free. I began to use my weekly allowance to collect 45s of the great soul musicians and spent nights dancing in my bedroom to the local soul radio station. More important, I learned that soul was not only an aspect of religion but also something that brought joy, authenticity, and creativity. I realized that there were experiences in life that were definitely good for the soul, and one of them was creative expression.

While we each come to appreciate and define soul in our own way, the soul has always been recognized, venerated, and cherished. It is most often defined as the immaterial essence, animating principle, or driving cause of one's life, a quality that kindles emotion and spirit. The idea of soul has permeated our lives for centuries, from shamanic soul retrieval to religious practices offering purification of the soul. Wisdom traditions around the world tell of soul illness, in which body, mind, and spirit are out of alignment with each other. We speak of loss of soul, a time when we lose touch with our true selves and our direction, intention, and meaning, or when we are not fulfilling our life purpose. The person who has experienced a loss of soul is unable to connect with others or make an inner connection to the self. Without the soul, one loses one's raison d'être and is profoundly alone.

Soul is, in a sense, the summation of the self, reflecting body and mind, ideas and perceptions, spirit and the world. It is the essence that signals us when we are not true to ourselves or when we have forgotten life's purpose because of trauma, emotional loss, physical illness, or unsatisfying relationships. It is equally the part of our being that helps us feel alive, reach down to the bones, and awaken ourselves to the goodness and gifts within each of us. Like James Brown, when we have a lot of soul, we have a zest for life, palpable energy, and a deep sense of well-being.

The soul is also viewed as a quality of consciousness and inner being. When we describe this aspect of soul, we often think of spirit, but these are two very different concepts. In simple terms, spirit is that which is transcendent, taking us beyond the self, while soul is our life energy and acts as part of a greater life force. It not only is at the center of being but is also that which connects us to other individuals, communities, nature, and the divine. We can share soul because its essence has no boundaries. Soul includes family, friends, the environment, and spirit. It opens up a dimension to experiencing life and self with depth, heart, and fellowship.

There are many ways to contact soul, but most often the soul's presence is awakened through some sort of spiritual practice. Meditation and prayer are but two of many ways that have been used to encounter soul throughout the world. While prayer certainly played a large role in my childhood and meditation has become a practice in my adult life, as an artist and therapist I also believe that art making is a practice that can awaken soul as much as spiritual techniques. Art is an authentic language of the soul and a mirror of the true nature of the soul's experience.

James Hillman equates soul with imagination, our potential to dream, fantasize, create, and form a mental image of something not present to the senses. Imagination can give us joy, hope, and pleasure; for this reason, it is central to our capacity to confront and deal with obstacles in life and to invent solutions to problems. In essence, imagination is both medicine for the soul and a wellness practice that helps us create new ways of seeing and being in the world.

Our ability to imagine is complemented by something uniquely human—our capacity to use imagination to create tangible visual images. Archeologists and anthropologists actually determine the existence of ancient human cultures by evidence of image making in the form of hand-crafted objects, decorative elements, sculptural forms, drawings, and paintings. Our need and drive to imagine and create images sets us apart from all other species. We are consistently drawn to creative expression to celebrate life's events and to make things that are special, just for the pleasure of it. While artists may create something extraordinary or unique through painting or sculpting, in day-to-day life we may dress in special clothes for important occasions, decorate our homes for holidays and celebrations, or create a special meal to commemorate an event. These are visual ways of making things special; embellishing and decorating our bodies, dwellings, and communities; and most important, celebrating ourselves as human beings capable of creative expression.

We humans intuited that art making was good for us in one way or another. I believe that our capacity to use our creative source for health and well-being is no different today. The miracle of our humanness is that we have the ability to create images with meaning. The simple act of making art nourishes the inner self and connects us with the outer world of relationships, community, and nature. It is a natural process of caring for the soul and experiencing it in all its dimensions.

DARK NIGHT OF THE SOUL:
THE CALL TO CREATIVE EXPRESSION

Each of us yearns to communicate experiences in such a way that others may know who we are and recognize our significance. But although our creative potential is always available to us, as an art therapist I have witnessed that it often takes an abrupt change in life circumstances to lead us to its reparative powers. It is the dark night of the soul that brings us to find a healing path. For this reason, the quest to recover one's soul is rarely ever consciously planned. The loss of a loved one, a medical emergency, or an emotional crisis are a few of the experiences that may startle us out of habitual patterns of existence. You may wake up one day to find that a good friend has died, that you have lost your job, or that you have been diagnosed with a serious illness and must make decisions about treatment while confronting your own mortality.

Although most people are not necessarily seeking a reconnection with soul when they first call to make an appointment with a doctor or therapist, the experience of being in distress often leaves them with wanting something more. Many years ago I was taught the soul's urgency and how it brings forth the need to create something from what seems senseless, random, and chaotic. Jean, a young woman in her mid-twenties, appeared, unannounced, in the doorway of my office late one afternoon. She had heard that I was an art therapist and told me that she had some drawings that she hoped I might like to see. Jean opened a large knapsack, and several sketchbooks spilled onto my desk; each one was completely filled with images— mostly crayon drawings and some collages she had made from scraps of paper and magazine clippings. As she opened each book to leaf through the pages, I could see that she was intensely interested in what I might have to say about her images. She also treated each drawing or collage with great care, love, and reverence.

When I asked her how she had come to fill so many sketchbooks with images, Jean told me that she had only recently felt compelled to make drawings. I wondered out loud if she thought there was any particular reason for this. She replied that she was having blackouts, periods of time when she could not remember what had happened. Sometimes she would find herself in her car several miles into a canyon road on the outskirts of town, not recalling how she had arrived there. Other times she would forget to go to work for several days in a row, then suddenly realize that she had not left her home for that time span. Following these experiences, she was often plagued with panic attacks followed by severe depression that kept her housebound for weeks at a time. These experiences not only were affecting her job and school performance but also caused her to fear that she was going insane. She was afraid that whatever was trying to "steal her soul" was succeeding and believed that art making was the only way to overcome what was happening to her.

While Jean's blackouts confused me, I was even more mystified by the images in her sketchbook. Some of the drawings looked like those of a young adult who had some basic skills and perhaps had done some drawing in high school or college. But many others seemed remarkably like the work of children of various ages. Many looked exactly like the scribbles of a toddler, others reflected the early depictions of a five-year-old, and still others seemed like artworks of an older child.

While I was happy to try to help Jean understand her images, I was reasonably sure that I was in over my head in other ways. Her blackouts and memory problems were troubling, and her panic attacks and depression needed evaluation and possibly medical intervention. I suspected that some trauma was behind her experiences and possibly had a connection to her drawings. I contacted a colleague, a family therapist who had experience working with survivors of trauma, for consultation. With Jean's agreement, we began to work together in weekly sessions in which he used a combination of hypnosis and family therapy techniques. During these sessions, I asked Jean to draw whatever surfaced in her mind's eye.

In the months that followed, we worked with Jean to help her discover the meaning of her images. What emerged slowly was that Jean had suffered severe abuse as child and was now struggling with dissociative identity disorder—a condition that results from years of early childhood trauma. Her dissociation allowed her to take on several different personalities, children and teenagers with memories of the abuse and neglect she experienced. When she engaged one of these personalities, she would draw in a style that reflected the age of the child or teenager who was present in her mind and body.

Through art expression Jean was able to uncover memories of her abuse and begin the long process of integrating experiences too horrible to speak out loud. Art images also became a way for Jean and me to begin to unravel the life story that she had buried deep within her in order to cope with the suffering of her childhood. While art helped Jean on her path to recovery, the road was not easy, and I was the first of many people to help her find her way through a maze of memories and stressful symptoms. Happily, many years later she no longer has the intrusive memories, panic attacks, or blackouts of the past, and now works as a physician's assistant. She has never given up image making and still makes crayon drawings and takes photographs of nature as a form of relaxation. Every few months I receive a letter from Jean with a drawing enclosed. Often it is one that she says has been created by one of her inner children and "colored especially for Cathy." She remains in touch with the creative imagination that she found within herself, as she says, "because drawing is still good for me and makes my soul happy."

I believe that Jean used art not only to soothe her soul but also, as she said in our first meeting, to save her soul. Art making was a lifeline, providing her with a sanctuary from frightening experiences that had become daily occurrences. The simple act of drawing or pasting pictures into her visual journals not only sustained her; it became a visual representation for the story of—and eventual recovery from—the abuse she experienced. Jean's intuition and sheer courage taught me about the strength of the human spirit as well as the soul's drive to well-being through creativity and imagination, even in the face of terror and personal devastation.

Witnessing Jean's image making and eventual recovery is one of the many creative journeys of individuals that have inspired me to look more deeply into how art reveals and heals, replenishes and restores, enlivens and renews. It appears as a remedy for those of us in search of balance, well-being, and wholeness. Whether I am in the presence of children from violent homes or adults facing life-threatening illnesses, or simply alone in my studio enjoying the colors of paint or the texture of clay, art is a constant agent of transformation and is indeed the soul's drive to health.

ART AS AN AWAKENING AGENT

A favorite story about the Buddha takes place during his wanderings through India shortly after his enlightenment. Several men who met him noticed that there was something wondrous about him. One asked, "Are you a god?" He answered, "No." Another asked, "Are you an angel?" "No," he replied. A third man asked, "Are you a magician?" Again, his answer was no. The men were confused by his responses and finally asked, "Well, what are you then?" He then answered, "I am awake."

How to awaken was the essence of what the Buddha taught. Spiritual practices such as meditation are forms of awakening. In a similar vein, art making is an awakening agent, one that is available to anyone and especially helpful in times of stress. People who are experiencing crisis or loss have discovered, often synchronistically, that art making can be a life-changing practice, even when one has had no formal art training.

Elizabeth Grandma Layton is an inspiring example of someone whose life was changed through the experience of art as awakener. Layton began to draw during her old age, without any previous training or experience, to help herself overcome thirty years of manic-depressive illness. According to Layton, electroshock treatments, lithium, and psychotherapy had failed to bring any lasting relief from her mental illness. Following the death of her son in 1976 when she was sixty-seven, Layton enrolled in a drawing class in a nearby college at her sister's suggestion. The only class available at that time was one in contour drawing—a technique in which one makes a line drawing of an object without looking at the paper on which one is drawing.

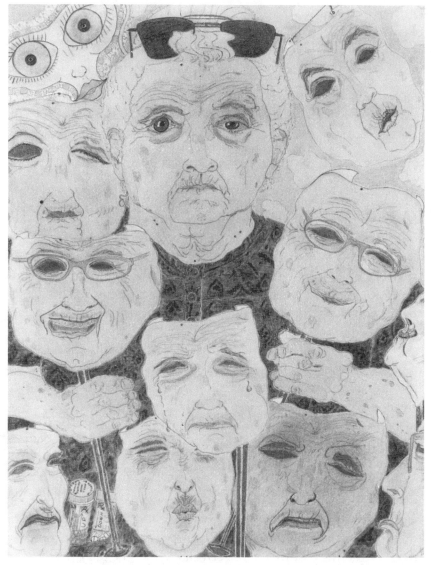

Masks, drawing by Elizabeth Layton during her recovery from depression.

Layton's instructor told her that if she had no other subject in mind to draw, she could simply draw herself. She took this advice and began creating a series of contour drawings that depicted every wrinkle, age spot, and aspect of her elderly body. But while completing these drawings, other ideas emerged in her work: concerns about society's treatment of the elderly, her own struggles with aging, and her experience with depression, grief, and loss. She began to feel her mood change, and her symptoms disappeared.

Layton never sold any of her more than one thousand drawings, fearing that the magic of the process would disappear, although she did give many of them to family, friends, and charity. Her work demonstrates that creativity is important throughout the life span and that feelings need to be expressed, whether through art or by other means, in order to be resolved. Through creative expression and imagination we naturally find ourselves developing new stories for life experiences and discover that we are awakened to something beyond pain, suffering, and illness.

HEART AND SOUL: ART AS PSYCHOTHERAPY

While creative expression is a powerful agent of awakening for the soul, art making is also a therapy for emotional pain and suffering. Layton used drawing as a way to grieve profound losses in her life, including the death of her son, and to confront her lifelong mood disorder. In my work as an art therapist, I have seen many other examples of art's powers to transform and repair psychological trauma.

Six-year-old Michael is a typical instance. On the first day I met with him at an outpatient trauma center, he silently drew an image of the fatal car accident that killed his parents. Michael had been in the car but was saved by his seatbelt and escaped with only minor physical injuries. In subsequent sessions I sat next to him on the floor, observing him as he repeatedly depicted the crash and the bodies of his parents, thrown through the front windshield. Gradually, I began to ask him if he could draw other memories of the accident and try to make an image of what he imagined death to be like. Although the tasks were difficult and tears welled in his eyes, he created a series of drawings of the ambulance coming to the accident scene, the police taking him to the station, a social worker who brought him to his grandmother's, and finally his parents in heaven. Michael's memories were painful, but the act of drawing helped him to grieve and to communicate his fears and anxieties in a way that words could not. He was able to illustrate the memories that had terrorized him each night, beginning the process of recovery and reparation from a profound loss.

Art's power as therapy for painful memories and emotions is equally potent for adults. One young woman with whom I worked was violently abused as a child by a stepparent. As a result, she ran away from home as a teenager and never contacted her family again. Her memories of the abuse and her grief over losing touch with her family became so pervasive that they began to intrude on her work, relationships, and joy of living. She was deeply depressed and tormented by physical symptoms, including severe pain and headaches. We decided that it might be helpful for her to give that pain a voice through color and shapes, by drawing the places in her body that hurt. For the first time in many years, the woman began to slowly release some of the inner suffering and anger she had been holding on to since leaving her family. While art making could not erase the abuse that she had experienced, giving her emotions a visual voice allowed her to reexperience the past in a way that helped to transform her sadness and despair into hope and trust.

Another family I met with was in crisis because of the recurrence of cancer in their teenage daughter. The daughter had been in remission and doing well when suddenly the cancer reappeared in her lungs and was diagnosed as inoperable. I asked the family to help me to understand through drawing what it was like for them as a family to live in such stressful circumstances. Using the metaphor of being marooned on a tropical island, they created a simple drawing together representing their sense of isolation. This group drawing expressed their grief and feelings of helplessness as the daughter's health slowly deteriorated. The visual symbol of an island brought up issues of separation, survival, adaptability, and courage, giving the parents and siblings a chance to share emotions that each had kept secret for fear of burdening the others. By the end of the session they had identified not only their strengths as a family but also ways to reach beyond their island to receive help and support from others.

These individuals' stories have one thing in common: the creative process of art making can unleash and transform a wounded heart. In each case, the emphasis was not on producing a finished work of art but rather on using the creative process to express the self, increase self-awareness, and give birth to a new story for one's life.

The idea of using art as therapy for emotional distress formally emerged in the early twentieth century. Sigmund Freud proposed a theory of how the unconscious expresses itself through the images of dreams and fantasies. During the same period, Carl Jung formulated the theory of the collective unconscious, a body of cross-cultural symbols and archetypes passed down through generations in the medium of art and mythology. While Freud was fascinated by primitive art and amassed an extensive collection, Jung had a personal interest in art and created his own drawings, paintings, and carvings throughout his life, recording and exploring his dreams in visual art. He believed that our hands know how to solve a problem with which the intellect has struggled in vain. Both Freud and Jung realized that language was not always adequate and that images, either in the form of art or in dreams, could provide wisdom and inner guidance that words alone could not.

During the last one hundred years the idea that creative visual expression was symbolic took hold, and psychiatrists and psychologists came to realize the importance of art as a reflection of our inner world of emotion. Art therapy, the use of the creative process for emotional restoration and healing, grew out of the idea that images are symbolic communications and that art making helps us to express and transform difficult life experiences. It has expanded our understanding of how image making and imagination help during the dark night of the soul, carrying forward the ancient knowledge of art's healing powers as well as the work of Freud and Jung. Artistic expression is one of our elemental tools for achieving psychological integration, a universal creative urge that helps us strive for emotional well-being.

BODY AND SOUL: ART AS MEDICINE

Art as a form of medicine for the body is an old tradition. Early Middle Eastern cultures used different colors of wool based on magical formulas for protection from disease, what would now be called preventive medicine or health maintenance. The native peoples of the American Southwest use sandpaintings to depict, then expunge illness, and symbolic totem animals are created to restore or strengthen psychological and spiritual health. I believe these artistic remedies for physical distress indicate that we humans naturally know what is good for us.

Today there is a resurgence of the arts at major medical centers, offering patients opportunities to create art, view the art of others, and experience artist-designed interiors. Patient-created art is enlivening hospital walls, and bed trays are filled with pens, paints, clay, and paper. We are learning that despite physical illness or debilitating medical treatment, the creative source within flourishes and people naturally reach for something within themselves that makes them feel whole even if pain and symptoms are not completely alleviated. Children undergoing chemotherapy or radiation work freely with crayons and paint; a teenager on dialysis often rifles through my art box to find the perfect color to match the sky outside the clinic window, unconscious of my presence or that of a nurse who is busily taking his blood pressure. Adults with cancer who have not touched art materials since they were children suddenly find themselves eager to participate in a weekly art group at local cancer support programs.

Forty-six-year-old Beth found the medicine of artistic expression eight years ago when she was first diagnosed with ovarian cancer. A nurse in an intensive care unit at a busy university medical center, she was reeling from the shock of sudden surgery, radiation treatments, and chemotherapy. When I first met her, Beth observed, "Everything around me has gone out of control. Everything but this sketchbook. This is where I can find some peace, escape, and control of my life."

As Beth adjusted to the realization that her body was seriously ill, she picked up a box of felt markers and began to draw. Like many people, Beth did not see herself as an artist but felt compelled to record her experiences in some way other than words alone. By the time I first met with her in my studio, she had already filled a large folder with drawings about her feelings, medical treatment, and struggles to make sense of her life as a person with a life-threatening illness. While she was lost in an hour or two of art making, she realized that she had less physical pain and nausea from chemotherapy and often emerged from a creative activity feeling more rested and less stressed.

Like Beth, others have experienced arts medicine for body and soul in time of crisis. Some say art making helps them to survive the devastation of illness and make sense of their experiences with cancer. Others are actually spiritually moved to make images—drawings, paintings, sculptures, photographs, quilts—to tell their stories and to record day-to-day experiences.

Physicians are recognizing and embracing the potential of art to heal patients in ways that medicine cannot. Bernie Siegel, whose work with people with cancer has influenced the holistic treatment of patients, has repeatedly said he wished all medical doctors would add a box of crayons to their diagnostic and therapeutic tools. After years of work as a surgeon, he found himself wanting to know how patients really saw their illness, doctor, and medical treatment. He knew that most people did not honestly express their emotions and fears of death to their doctors. Through asking his patients to make simple crayon drawings, Siegel began to learn their deepest worries, what they saw as helpful to their well-being, and what they believed about their doctor, surgery, radiation, and chemotherapy. The soul's palette, often through expressions as simple as stick figures and primitive marks on paper, reflected the true experience of both physical illness and the mind's fears.

John Graham-Pole, a pediatric oncologist in Florida, became an artist out of his need to find compassion and meaning in his own work with children whose lives were threatened by cancer. He began writing poetry to make sense of the suffering he witnessed daily and ended up awakening to the value of the arts in creating humanity and community in the midst of pain and suffering. This discovery inspired him to found an arts medicine program at his hospital to help patients reclaim their innate creativity during the crisis of illness. Picture in your mind a room next to the nurses' station where the young patients can gather while they are waiting to be seen by a doctor or receiving their intravenous medication or a blood transfusion. The room is filled wall-to-wall, wall-to-ceiling, with paintings, drawings, and collages. This gallery spills out into the hall into what John calls the hospital's version of a wax museum, a collection of body-tracings in loving connection to one another. The ceilings on the way to surgery rooms are covered with images so that young patients have something creative to see on the way to surgery. Through the unit, artists, students, and volunteers come to help children and their families create art at bedside, in waiting rooms, and in hallways.

Beth's inspirational drive to creativity at the time of serious illness, Bernie's realization that images reflect a deeper sense of self, and John's vision of hospital as studio are a few of the many stories of how the soul's palette tends to our bodies and minds when we are confronted with physical illness, disability, or death. Art as medicine simply is the manifestation of the soul's drive toward health.

COMMUNITY SOUL-UTIONS

Over the last several centuries the art world has become a place of commodities, placing monetary value on what we come to embrace as great art. Many artists have sought something beyond commercial value in their search for the meaning of artistic expression. Suzi Gablik refers to this as the "reenchantment of art," a return to the tradition of spirit in art as a reflection of self and the arts as a powerful force in the life of individuals, communities, and the world.

Historically and cross-culturally, artists were core leaders of their communities and often assumed the role of shaman. In this identity, artists were not seen as individuals in pursuit of personal expression but instead were acknowledged as the creative source of insight and wisdom for the collective group. Artists had a mission to engage others to join in using the arts as a tool for individual and collective change and as a way of realizing the deep connectedness to one another and the world.

The use of art as a spiritual and transformative practice within communities is currently experiencing a revival. The city of Lynn in northeastern Massachusetts has a crime rate that is 50 percent higher

than the national average, and high substance abuse, teenage preg-
nancy, and school dropout rates. It is a racially diverse community
with Latino, Cambodian, and African American residents, and a growing Russian population, all of whom are at the lower economic or
poverty level. In the midst of Lynn's Central Square, a group of artist-
therapists, led by Mary Flannery and Kit Jenkins, took their dream
of a creative oasis from urban problems and envisioned Raw Art
Works (RAW), a community-based art therapy program confronting
the needs of children, inner-city families, and incarcerated youth.

Flannery and Jenkins's idea of art making as a "soul-ution" to the
community's problems was more than successful. Soon the two women
found themselves in collaboration with the very youth who were RAW's
first clients and expanded the boundaries of their original vision. These
teens became mentors for others, carrying forth their enthusiasm and
understanding of how art transforms lives to those in the community
who are in need of the creative process. As a result, the initial vision
for an inner-city art therapy program has become an alternative to gang
involvement, and among these young mentors, all have stayed in

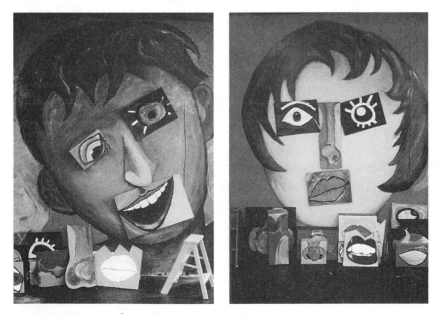

Interactive Portraits from the RAW Art Works
"Colors Have Feelings, Too" exhibit.

school, 80 percent have applied to college, and everyone feels safe, successful, and connected to the community.

Flannery and Jenkins are visionaries who represent a growing movement in the arts to take creativity to soup kitchens, public housing, incarceration facilities, clinics, and inner-city schools, and into people's homes. The need for creative expression is finding its way into the larger terrains where healing must take place: institutions, neighborhoods, cities, and even the planet. It is the manifestation of the soul's palette as a creative force to restore, replenish, and renew community.

Artists are bringing wellness to the souls of communities in other ways. In metropolitan areas, art is being infused into the tenuous worlds of the homeless, drug abusers, and street gangs. Public art projects focus on helping communities create spaces that express not only aesthetic qualities but also images that provide emotional balance, well-being, and health for those living there. Art making is being used as a catalyst to bring delinquent teens and police forces together and to facilitate dialogue about violence, shootings, and substance abuse. Community soul-utions are a growing trend around the world as Doctors Without Borders, therapists, artists, and volunteers are offering artistic expression to children in worn-torn Bosnia-Herzegovina and other disaster areas.

The soul's palette has reached the workplace, where creativity can not only change the individual but also transform companies, agencies, and institutions. RAW has extended its services to the corporate world, to help employees think outside of the box, encourage honest and effective communication, and cultivate personal strengths. Artists are impacting the workplace in other ways that touch the souls of corporations, institutions, and agencies. Regina Kelley, a sculptor, brings collaborative art-making experiences to medical professionals and hospice staff with the goal of developing healing art installations. In designing one sculpture installation, she asked each staff person—doctors, nurses, support staff, and janitors—to make a small sculpture depicting what he or she did to relax after work. She combined the pieces in a bronze column that stands in the garden of the facility. The presence of this collaborative work reminds the staff members of their connection to their community and what contributes to their own personal healing.

A NEVER-ENDING CREATIVE SOURCE

The soul's palette is so many things: an agent of transformation, a therapy for the psyche, a salve for body and mind, and a remedy for the ills of individuals, communities, and the world. Visual images, whether made of canvas or clay, produce profound physical and emotional benefits and are an unending source of inner knowledge. They are a way to bare our souls, to get to the soul of the matter, to go on a soul search. Like an artist's palette that contains an infinite spectrum of colors and choices for creating, our soul's palette is a boundless source of wisdom and wellness.

A creative act is one that invokes imagination, making the invisible visible. It reflects what is inside of us, parts of the self that are more authentically conveyed with images than with words. One could call that an internalized image of oneself, but in its simplest sense, it is as close as we get to seeing our souls.

The miracle of the soul's palette remains alive within you. Even if you have neglected it since early childhood, you have nothing to worry about—it's still there, fully intact. It is not limited by your age, physical condition, or art training. It is connected to the creative instincts you were born with, and it is your life force, energy, zest for life. It does not require that you produce a finished work of art worthy of display in a museum, but it does ask you to be authentic, and it is called forth by simply being yourself.

Your creative source is the authentic reflection of soul, in all its infinite colors, forms, and symbols. In the chapters that follow you will learn the many ways you can reclaim your creative source and tap the wisdom of your soul's palette. Even if you consider yourself to be a "non-artist," you can experience the healing journey of self-discovery, reparation, and transformation that is nourished and enhanced through the process of taking pen or paintbrush in hand. Your imagination, dreams, visions, and creative urges are the soul's promptings to health and to a rediscovery of who you are and all that you can be.

Creativity as a Healing Force

hile artistic creativity is a therapy for mind, body, and soul, there are specific reasons why it is good for your overall well-being. This chapter explains why art is a healing force and how you can begin to bring it into your life through creative art activities and deepen its powers through transformative practices.

This chapter also sets the stage for two concepts that are repeated throughout the book: creative activities and transformative practices. Creative activities are exercises that will help you to develop and enhance your creative powers, tap your imagination's healing potential, and access and use imagery for personal growth. Transformational practices are long-term creative experiences designed to deepen and enhance the potential of art in your life. Both can help you to make art an integral part of health maintenance.

THE ART OF HEALING

To understand just how art heals, it is important to first understand what healing means. The best explanation of healing that I have ever heard is given by Michael Lerner, Commonweal Cancer Program, in

Bolinas, California, who offers a fundamental distinction between healing and curing. This distinction is rooted in one of the greatest and oldest traditions in wellness among tradition cultures, yet is not fully recognized by mainstream Western medicine today.

Lerner explains that a cure is a treatment that removes all evidence of the disease and eliminates all evidence of disease. A cure is what the physician hopes to bring to the patient. Healing, in contrast, is an inner process through which a person becomes whole, the sense of being intact and undiminished, and can take place on physical, emotional, or spiritual levels. In a physical sense, a wound or a broken bone may heal; on an emotional level, there may be recovery from childhood abuse or the death of a loved one; and on a spiritual level, there may be a deeper reconnection with God or nature, or an experience of inner peace or oneness with the world.

Although curing and healing are different, wisdom traditions tell us that they are also interconnected with regard to health and well-being. When a tribal medicine woman prescribes an herbal remedy or a physician stitches a wound, both are engaging in therapy to speed recovery. But if the capacity to heal is not present, both the medicine woman and the physician know that their efforts may not be effective. With a more holistic philosophy emerging in contemporary medicine, we are becoming more aware of the role of our inner healing capacities, which support the recuperative powers of body and mind.

The miracle of healing, however, goes beyond curing and takes place when curing is impossible. In cases where it is no longer possible for the body to recover from cancer or other illness, healing still continues on emotional and spiritual levels. Medicine does not yet know whether a patient's efforts to heal have significant impact on *length* of life, but it is obvious that healing—becoming whole—has a powerful impact on the *quality* of life.

The experience of becoming whole, while very real to the individual, is an unseen process. Art and healing are intimately connected because it is through imagination and image making that you can stimulate and witness the process of becoming whole. Even if you already are satisfied with your life, relationships, health, and work, your creative source brings you closer to who you are and reflects your inner being in ways that other forms of healing cannot.

CREATIVE EXPRESSION AS A
WELLNESS PRACTICE

Thomas Edison predicted that the doctor of the future will give no medicine but will interest patients in prevention of disease and self-care. Unlike traditional medical paradigms that focus on the treatment of illness, wellness is a philosophy of promoting health and preventing disease. It is something that must be practiced to be achieved and is also a personal belief about what health is. In my experience, people with disease or disability report nonetheless that they perceive themselves as having an inner sense of health, a deeper recognition of well-being than merely physical. What is even more interesting is that when people have a sense of wellness, they often live beyond medical expectations (in the case of disease) and experience a greater joy and enthusiasm about life itself.

There are many ways that we can find wellness—intimate relationships, social contacts, spirituality or religion, nature, and service to others have all been shown to increase our belief that we are well. Ranked high among these experiences is creative expression—using one's imagination, making images, and enjoying artworks as a spectator. Our ability to imagine and communicate through visual means is a wellness practice that is natural to us, one that humankind has engaged for well-being throughout recorded history. In fact, the creative expression—painting, crafts, decoration, and rituals—was probably used as a way to experience wellness and to increase our sense of health in both good times as well as periods of stress, pain, or suffering.

Imagery and imagination have been recognized forms of complementary therapy that have the capacity to produce positive physical changes in the body, enhance emotional resilience, and cope with life's difficult moments. Herbert Benson, a pioneer in the field of complementary medicine—treatment that complements traditional (allopathic) medicine—explains that images can help us achieve "remembered wellness." How we imagine our experiences and what we believe about them have a powerful effect on our sense of well-being. Our internalized images can actually activate brain connections that produce symptoms—but fortunately they can also alleviate ailments, pain, and distress. If we use our imaginative capacities to produce imagery of what it was like to be without symptoms, we can remember wellness and increase our immediate sense of well-being.

Creative activities are being used in health-care programs because of their numerous benefits to overall wellness, including stress reduction and relaxation, improvement of blood pressure, heart rate, and respiration, improving mood and outlook, and increased capacity to communicate feelings about symptoms. These benefits come not only from engaging in the artistic process but also from exposure to works of art, carefully designed interiors, and the images of nature. Since ancient times, humans have understood that the imagery of nature and environments is crucial for healing. In Delphi, temples of great beauty were designed as healing sanctuaries set in magnificent natural sites. More than one hundred years ago Florence Nightingale, the English pioneer of nursing as a profession for women, observed that beautiful objects, especially of a brilliancy of color, had a palliative effect on her patients. Impressed by the power of images to induce wellness, she proclaimed that they not only healed the mind but also had a physical effect on the body and were means of recovery. What the Greeks and Nightingale discovered is now becoming commonplace to hospitals, clinics, hospices, and rehabilitative centers.

Creative activities are known to enhance brain functioning and structure, alleviate depression, and give rise to alpha wave patterns typical of restful alertness, the relaxed but aware state found in meditation. The frontier of psychoneuroimmunology—the study of the interrelationship of mind and body, behavior and health—has demonstrated that imagery may be an important factor in self-healing and may even have a far-reaching influence on others. Numerous studies, such as those described by Larry Dossey, M.D., have shown that prayers and positive intentions on behalf of others help speed recovery of patients who did not even know they were being prayed for. Our mental imagery has a similar potential in directing our own bodies to relax, increase blood flow, dilate veins, reduce heart rate, and stimulate the immune system.

Art making may actually be a fountain of youth, particularly when age is viewed as a state of mind and spirit rather than body alone. I have always been deeply moved by a photograph of artist Henri Matisse in his old age drawing and painting in his studio. Even when he was confined to his bed in the last days of life, he had someone attach a piece of charcoal to a long stick and would draw on a paper placed above him on the ceiling. He also created collages, works of brilliantly colored paper cutouts arranged spontaneously, but with an unfailing eye for design, on a canvas surface. Matisse's drive to express his artistic imagination was exceptionally strong, but I believe that his story holds a message for all of us: creativity is a healing response to disability or failing health.

Deepak Chopra observes that the single most important factor for health and well-being is that we make something creative from our existence. Evidence from neurology and evolutionary psychology increasingly suggests that the arts play an important role in our abilities to think, problem-solve, and remember. Images, whether in the form of art making, imagination, or dreams, naturally help maintain and stimulate our minds and bodies. Our creative source actually extends the life span and may be just as important to health maintenance as good nutrition, exercise, and medical care. It keeps us vital and in connection with life in ways that other forms of medicine for the body cannot.

Artistic expression is an instinctive practice that ultimately comes from one's own innate being. Using one's own creativity is somewhat similar to the practice of homeopathy, which stimulates the body's own resources to treat illness. A homeopath, in essence, seeks a remedy based on the individual's unique constellation of physical and psychological symptoms. Artistic expression has a similar capacity because it comes from within us, working with and stimulating our own means to resolve and heal the problem.

USING YOUR SENSES AND
FEELING YOUR THOUGHTS

Part of what makes the creative process of art making different from other forms of healing is the use of the senses to express, experience, and communicate. It involves vision, touch, movement, sound, and even smell. Images translate stories more tangibly than words because they not only contain ideas but make them both seen and felt.

Externalizing your experiences, even through a simple drawing, is a powerful self-transformer. Recently, research on traumatized individuals has shown us that experiences such as coloring with a crayon, even scribbling, have far-reaching effects on how we feel and how we see our life experiences.[1] Art expression can renew a connection to emotion for an individual who has been traumatized and mobilize creativity as a healing force for recovery and well-being.

Expressing our experiences through drawing actually helps us to express our feelings verbally as well—more so than if we were only asked to talk about them. This is especially true if we have experienced a profound crisis in our lives, when words are difficult or unavailable. I recently worked with seven-year-old Bobby, who witnessed the accidental shooting of a classmate in gang-related gunfire just a few blocks from Bobby's home. After the incident, Bobby understandably became withdrawn and depressed in the weeks following the death of his friend.

When Bobby sat down in my art and playroom, he seemed uninterested in the toys and games and sat looking down into his lap. I asked him if he liked to draw, and he mumbled a quiet yes. I told him I had a scribble-drawing game that I thought he would be good at and placed a large piece of white paper on the desk at which we both sat. I started the drawing game by asking Bobby to follow my pen scribbling across the paper with his pen for a short time until the paper was filled with lines. I then asked him to look at the scribble we made and to use the drawing materials to make a picture using the lines.

Bobby spent the next twenty minutes carefully creating a series of pictures from the scribble: a car running over a person, a man shooting another man, and a fire consuming a building. It was easy to see that he was focused on themes of danger and destruction. Like many children who are exposed to violence, he was carrying vivid images in his head but had had no way of speaking about them. Drawing became an outlet for the fears he had suffered since witnessing the shooting.

In subsequent meetings Bobby used drawing to create different solutions to the themes he had expressed in the scribble drawing, such as how a person could avoid being run over by the car and what to do if someone was caught in a burning building. Most important, he portrayed his feelings of fear, anxiety, and guilt about what had happened to his friend. In our last meeting, Bobby said that he was happy that he could now talk to his parents about his feelings when he was apprehensive or sad. Art helped Bobby to communicate his feelings by reexperiencing what had happened through his own creative resources.

When asked to draw a memory, we are usually able to give far more verbal details when we express ourselves in images than through talking alone. It is as if the drawing stimulates something inside us that helps us to generate ideas, associations, and perceptions about our experiences. This seems to be particularly true for emotionally laden events such as trauma or profound loss. Artistic expression may actually increase memory retrieval, help us to organize our stories, and prompt us to tell more than we would with words.

Images are the midwives between experience and language. The miracle of image making, even a rudimentary scribble or doodle, is that it helps birth a story that holds countless memories and emotions. Through a single drawing or image, no matter how simple, we can express and contain multiple feelings, relationships, and hours of narrative—and, most important—visually translate our experiences on behalf of our souls.

GOING WITH THE FLOW AND BECOMING MINDFUL

A young woman with severe arthritis told me something insightful while she was completing a clay sculpture one afternoon in my studio. She said, "Making art helps me to slip off my disease for a while." This slipping off is one of art making's most remarkable qualities, one that actually alters our experience of who we are in the present moment. It allows us to reach a state of consciousness where we are no longer individuals with problems, pain, or suffering but beings who experience a sense of oneness through surrender to the creative process.

Shamans claim that there is a deeper dimension of reality where there is no time and space and the laws of nature do not apply in the usual ways. In the way of the shaman, this is the realm of healing. It seems the young woman in my studio was experiencing just that—

entry into a place where physical limitations do not matter. In this place she was not present to her body's pain and swollen joints, and her self-identification as a sick person did not exist.

The experience of being fully and deeply engaged in art making is an example of what psychologist Mihaly Csikszentmihalyi calls being in a state of "flow." The flow state is similar to that of meditation because it involves being both mindful and absorbed in the present moment. You may have observed how musicians lose themselves in their performance, or perhaps you have personally experienced the suspension of time that occurs when you are completely involved in gardening or in deep conversation with a friend. In this state of mind one becomes one with the process or activity with which one is engaged. Philosophers, scientists, and researchers agree that flow is a desirable state to be in, for its mental, emotional, and physical rewards are many.

Csikszentmihalyi says that flow is also about finding meaning in a particular activity, in a profession, or, if one is really fortunate, in life. In such cases, worry drops away, pain is absent, and you are at one with what you are doing. For example, if you are painting and you suddenly realize to your surprise that you've been working for three hours when it felt like ten minutes, then you have been in a flow state. This altered state of consciousness is sustained and deepened by the process of creating forms, working with colors, and developing images. Creative work is a natural flow-inducer that helps us to shut out chaos, focus our energies, and experience exhilaration. The seemingly simple moments of painting, drawing, or crafting are powerful gateways to catching the wave known as flow.

Flow experiences naturally also involve mindfulness—being fully awake to the present moment. Just as mindfulness meditation (the practice of calm awareness as thoughts enter our field of attention in the present) can help us tune down our stress and refresh our physical and mental being, art making and imaginative activities can have the same effect. When we become deeply engaged in art making, our minds may lose touch with the boundaries of self and other. Creative imagination insists that we give ourselves over to what we are doing with our hands, head, heart, and soul. In the process, we become mindful of the here and now.

TRANSCENDING SELF AND TOUCHING SPIRIT

Buddhism teaches us that the present moment contains the possibility for all things, including liberation from *samsara*, the world of suffering. When I have brought art making to the bedside of seriously ill children and adults, I have witnessed the potential of being in the present moment to free those suffering from their pain. They discover that they can often rise above illness, fears, and anxieties while engaged in artistic expression. These moments are, in a sense, experiences of transcendence, of liberation from samsara, and of going beyond one's illness to more fully enjoy and experience life.

The psychologist Abraham Maslow has suggested that when people's basic needs are satisfied—for food, shelter, and security—only then do they show a strong drive toward self-expression and the transcendent function of human nature. Satisfaction of basic needs allows creativity to emerge and flourish. But this is not always the case, especially when the soul's drive to care for itself is tested by life's most adverse conditions.

There are numerous examples, many in recent times, that illustrate how the will to create transcends all other needs, including food, shelter, and safety. Perhaps the most powerful example of the transcendent function of art took place at the Nazi concentration camp of Theresienstadt. This was supposed to be a model camp, which outsiders were shown to demonstrate to the world that Germany was treating concentration camp residents with respect and humanity. While living conditions were slightly better at Theresienstadt than at other camps, basic provisions were lacking, and people were regularly taken to their deaths at Auschwitz and other extermination sites or died within the camp under harsh and inhuman conditions.

The arts were nevertheless considered a priority by the residents, despite the harshness and cruelty of daily life. I was deeply touched while speaking with a survivor of the camp who told of a young artist who later was deported from Theresienstadt and killed by the Nazis. All people who were sent to Theresienstadt were given a list of items to pack for the move, things such as a bedroll, clothing, and cooking utensils. The artist instead filled his fifty-kilogram allowance with paints, brushes, paper, and canvas. He risked punishment and possible death through this action, but for him, art making was as necessary to survival as a coat, shoes, or knives and forks.

Others, including hundreds of children whose art survived as a legacy from the camp, transcended the loss of homes and possessions, illness, and constant confrontation with death through creative work. Art became a strategy for survival, in and of itself, providing a way to imagine happier circumstances or a memory of one's home. The vast amount of art (now housed in the Jewish Museum in Prague and the U.S. Holocaust Museum in Washington, D.C.), along with music and theater produced at Theresienstadt, is an impressive testimony to art's power to transcend and elevate the spirit regardless of hardship or adversity.

In more recent times, we have witnessed how people use art to rise above violence. The city of Sarajevo has been transformed from a beautiful European city to a war zone, the target of constant shelling and sniper fire. Despite these circumstances, its residents continued to express themselves through art and enjoyed music and theater, even while undergoing physical hardships such as lack of safe shelters and food. They persisted in maintaining orchestras and choirs and holding concerts. At one point, they turned a destroyed theater into an exhibition space for art created out of materials from the city's destruction.

Today, in neighboring Serbia, children in refugee camps are fearful that they may never see their families again. Some draw burning houses, bombs exploding, and broken, bloody bodies on the ground, a record of what they have witnessed on a daily basis. Others, no less experienced with death and destruction, paint sunflowers and daisies, bright blue skies, and golden sun rays shining down on houses and gardens. While reality bodes a grim future, many of these children try to create what they imagine life could be, demonstrating the resilience of the human spirit and the power of creativity to take us beyond chaos, hopelessness, and despair.

Experiences similar to those of the people of Theresienstadt, Sarajevo, and Serbia are played out in individual lives every day, with details perhaps less dramatic but nonetheless life-threatening and adverse. I witness countless individuals with cancer or HIV use art expression to overcome the effects of illness and to momentarily transcend their circumstance of being a cancer patient or a person with AIDS. Children hospitalized with serious injuries, leukemia, or severe burns, despite high fevers, infections, and fatigue, are eager to open my art box filled with pencils, colored papers, and glitter and make an image for their parent or for a nurse on the unit. For the time they are engaged in the process of making, creating, forming, and constructing, disabilities and pain are not a factor. Art making continually satisfies something deep inside us and, at the same time, places us beyond ourselves. Humanity's drive to self-express through art is a powerful and compelling need that often supersedes basic necessities.

BECOMING AN AUTHORITY AND MAKING MEANING

The examples just mentioned illustrate that the very act of drawing, painting, or constructing can be a personally empowering experience in contrast to life's tragedies. Even in daily life we feel that something, to a greater or lesser degree, in life is beyond our control. When more serious crises such as illness or loss occur, we may feel that the world has become chaotic, unjust, and senseless. At these times, we may turn to spiritual beliefs, prayer, or ritual—or to less desirable ways to calm the soul, through drugs, alcohol, overeating, or the numbing trance of staring at a television screen.

Ellie, a woman in her mid-twenties, began making art after several years of struggling with a major illness that debilitated both body and spirit. She developed pelvic inflammatory disease as a result of an intrauterine contraceptive device, but for months she did not know why she had fever, extreme pain, and exhaustion. When she was finally diagnosed, she was put on antibiotics that caused a severe drug reaction and almost killed her. For two years after, she continued to live with daily pain and, as she said, became a prisoner of her illness.

One day a friend brought her a large Mexican Talavera ceramic plate as a gift. Its colors and lively patterns intrigued her, and she got out a few marking pens and began to draw the designs on a notepad. Soon she was drawing more fanciful images, some from her imagination and others of landscapes, bowls of fruit, and flowers. When Ellie first came to my art therapy practice, she said she knew one certain truth about why art heals: "When I am drawing, I am in charge. Not even this illness can control me while I making pictures." She never experienced pain or fatigue while creating her drawings; her disease had no power or authority in her creative realm, and she was no longer its prisoner during those moments.

Art provides an active process that lets us choose materials, style, and subject matter, play freely with colors, lines, and forms with no rules, and create whatever we want. The creative source asks that each of us become our own authority on self-expression. While art historians and critics may dictate what the definition of great art is, it is only we ourselves who dictate what authentic creative expression can be. We also are the sole authority on how it is made and what it means, because art's medicine relies on us to define its images, symbols, and visual messages.

Medical intuitive and neuroscientist Mona Lisa Schultz explains the importance of creating meaning through one's inner intuitive resources, particularly when facing crisis or illness. She developed her own intuitive skills as a result of years of suffering from a sleep disorder that required several trials of medication in attempt to treat her condition. The side effects of the medication created mental confusion and left her to rely on her creative intuition rather than her then-jumbled intellect. Schultz came to realize that when the body demands one's attention because of illness or stress, it uses symbols to communicate its wisdom. The challenge becomes to be open to receiving this intuition and to have the courage to explore its meaning, authentically and creatively. It is through this process that meaning is known and healing occurs.

Images are a central source of meaning-making because they flow from your inner creative authority, the soul's palette. In this sense, artistic expression is always autobiographical and it inevitably tells the story of your life in all its dimensions—feelings, thoughts, experiences, memories, values, and beliefs. In the process of making these visible through image, you are offered a way to make meaning and an opportunity to transform that meaning into a deeper understanding of your life.

FINDING THE TRUTH WHILE
ENJOYING THE MYSTERY

Bernie Siegel says that the most important form of communication is visual and that our dreams, visions, and drawings speak the truth to us. Seeing countless patients' drawings of their illnesses and their medical treatment, he knows that their truths are only told to him through their images. Rachel Naomi Remen, also a physician who works with seriously ill individuals, offers another view of why imagery helps us find the truth. She describes imagery as the language of the unconscious and a way in which the unconscious parts of us are able to speak to our conscious selves. Remen makes the following analogy: If you are in France, she says, you need to learn to speak French in order to communicate. Similarly, if you are undertaking an inner voyage of healing, you must learn to use the language of dreams, poetry, art, religion, and myth to seek and to understand your personal truth.

Many years ago I worked with an adolescent girl whose grandfather had died after a prolonged illness. She was very close to her grandfather but was not allowed to see him in the hospital before he died and felt great sadness that she had not had a chance to say goodbye to him. She was depressed and felt incomplete and unfinished with their relationship.

One day she came into my office with a small painting she had created on notebook paper earlier that day, an image of a powerful dream she'd had the night before. In the dream her grandfather appeared in a large chair surrounded by all of his relatives, children, and grandchildren, with her sitting to his right. He gave everyone a blessing and told her that he would be leaving her and that he realized that she would be all right now. She then saw a reindeer come down from the sky and lead her grandfather away. She was surprised by what she described as a wonderful feeling of peace this dream gave her but also puzzled by the appearance of the reindeer. Despite a sense of confusion, she felt comforted by the image of the reindeer and was able to put aside much of her grief over the loss of her beloved grandparent.

A week later she brought back her small painting along with a symbol dictionary she had found in her high school library. She had

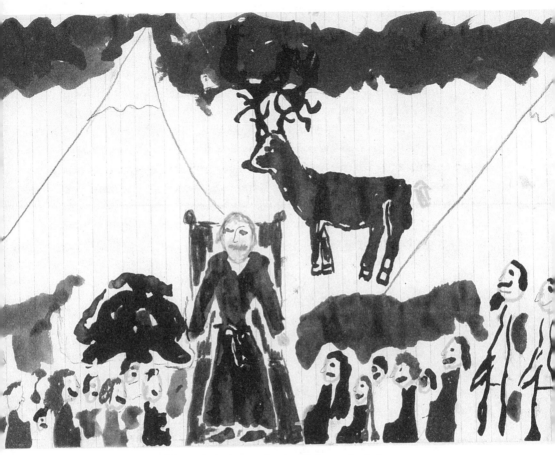

A dream painting of the artist's deceased grandfather and reindeer.

discovered a section of the dictionary on reindeers and what they have symbolized throughout history. To both her joy and surprise, the book explained that reindeers served as guides and often came to transport humans from earth to heaven. This description made sense of the lingering and mysterious element of her dream. From that day onward, she was able to resolve the crisis of her grandfather's passage and find consolation in the truth her dream conveyed.

Art indeed offers us another way of seeking the truth—through the inner realities of our feelings, experiences, beliefs, sensations, and perceptions. But unlike language, the primary form of communication in most cultures, imagination and artistic expression really have no grammar, syntax, or sentence structure. Art is not limited by reason, rules, or logic. On the one hand, art does communicate our truths; on the other, there is an inherent mystery to the source and content of art's imagery. Part of the healing and transformative possibilities of the soul's palette is that we may never fully or consciously know the complete meaning of the images we generate. The miracle of the creative adventure is that even though we never completely understand our encounters with truths through imagery, we still experience these truths on deeper levels. And even when we believe we have fully exhausted the meanings of our images, the mystery continues, because images are never completely understood. Their mysterious healing powers are continuously revealed to us as long as we have need of them.

AN EQUAL OPPORTUNITY EXPERIENCE

I often tell people in my workshops or therapy sessions to consider art making an "EOE"—in the jargon of the workplace, an equal opportunity experience. That is, anyone can engage in art making, even with minimal technical skill; the power of artistic expression lies in one's own investment and satisfaction in the process. What is truly extraordinary about the soul's palette is that you need no special talent, no drawing lessons, and no previous experience with art to begin using and benefiting from it. When you simply express yourself through images from a place of authenticity, your natural creative ability is automatically activated. The images you make—no matter in what form, content, or style—guide, support, motivate, activate, and ensoul the potential for well-being within you.

Although artistic imagination exists naturally in all of us, there are ways to cultivate it in order to get the most health-giving benefits from it. Over many years of facilitating people's experiences with art, I have found that there are two ways to incorporate artistic creativity into one's life. If we have limited time to engage in art expression, we can include art it as a short-term activity from time to time. To get the deepest, most long-lasting benefits, we can establish it in our lives as a long-term, transformational practice.

CREATIVE ACTIVITIES

Suppose you just want to experience art making on occasion as a form of relaxation, self-care, or personal satisfaction. In this case, it may be more feasible for you to learn more about simple activities you can enjoy in your spare time, alone or with friends or family. These experiences may inspire you to think more about the potential of art and imagination and to bring it into your life in new ways.

Throughout the rest of this book there are suggestions for activities that you can use to capitalize on the health-giving qualities of images every day and at any time. The wonder of the soul's palette as a source of wellness is that it includes not only making images but also using imagination and even witnessing images. I believe that making one's own images is the best way to get art's medicine, but experiencing images in other ways is also potent. Using the mind's eye to dream, to fantasize, to solve problems, and to take one beyond oneself is a wonderful way to engage art's power for personal well-being.

Viewing images on a regular basis, whether in the form of going to an art gallery, a well-designed space, or on a walk in nature, has the potential to enhance our sense of wellness. There are many people in this world who don't paint but who go to see and enjoy the paintings of others, and those who don't know how to use a potter's wheel who buy well-crafted bowls for their aesthetic beauty. Art stimulates both those who make it and those who witness it. Creating, imagining, and witnessing all instill within you a new sensibility about how you experience yourself and the world.

Creative activities are designed to introduce you to your inner artist and creative source, to help you express yourself through drawing, paint, clay, and collage, and to generally get your imagination flowing. You can experiment with these activities in the order they are presented in the book, skip those that don't interest you, or return to the activities that you enjoy when you want to reintroduce yourself to the ideas in this book. Think of activities that you find pleasure in repeating as old friends that can be called upon to enliven your world, bring you joy, relieve your stress, and express something new about yourself.

If you already identify yourself as an artist, the creative activities in this book may give you a jump start on a new way of working as an artist. Remember, these activities are not like lessons you may have learned in art classes at school. They ask you to take a different perspective on creative work, one that nourishes the self and cares for the soul. They also request that you create in an authentic way, without a preconceived notion of how art "should" be made, but rather to find your own personal way of making images. If you consider yourself to be a non-artist, it is important that you undertake these activities without a sense of self-judgment or censorship. (More about how to get started in seeing yourself as an artist is presented in the next chapter.)

TRANSFORMATIONAL PRACTICES

For those readers who want to go further and make the healing potentials of creativity a central part of life, this book includes transformational practices to stimulate that journey. Transformation is a process that involves positive, long-term change, and practice is the seedbed where the miracle of transformation takes place. There are numerous non-art traditions in the world that are grounded in transformational practices. Daily meditation, prayer, and service to others induce transformation in us over time. Exercise, good nutrition, and other health disciplines are also ways to promote change. When artistic expression becomes a regular part of our lives, it too can be a practice that brings both a deeper experience of well-being and a potential for profound changes in many parts of our lives.

Wisdom traditions see practice as a path or journey. The Chinese tradition of the Tao teaches that the path of practice is never-ending: the more we learn, the more there is to learn. In knowing, we create a need to know more. In art, the more we create, the more we can and want to create. In Buddhist philosophy, practice is sometimes viewed as a stream or river. This metaphor invokes the idea that there is a current already present to guide your journey. You need only decide to enter the river, and in doing so, you will be a different person. Even if at some point in time you decide to step out of the current, you will take some of its power with you.

The following example may inspire you to consider art making as a transformational practice in your life. For more than a decade, I have served as a facilitator for an arts and wellness group for women who are long-term survivors of cancer. When we first established the group, the majority of participants in the initial sessions jokingly complained that they were not artists and could not draw a straight line. But each group member was willing to take a risk and try her hand at drawing, painting, collage, sculpture, and photography during the eight-week course of our meetings.

Gradually, many of these women from the original group managed to shed their initial fears and doubts about art making and about their conceptions of artist. The transformations are apparent: for some, the idea that being an artist was impossible is now a distant memory, and they have embraced the creative source within as a regular part of life. For others, the practice of making art has broadened their personal lives; they are regular attendees at the latest exhibition at the art center, take classes at the local art school, or make time for art projects with their children. One even became an arts activist of sorts, starting fund-raising projects for community arts programs for the homeless, indigent, and elderly.

Art making as a transformational practice entails taking things at a slower pace and going deeper into the creative process and image work. It means turning to art on a regular basis in your life, not just as a treat for special occasions. But you don't have to wait until you have learned everything to begin a practice. Start where you are right now and enter the river.

THE IN-BETWEEN PATH

Unless being an artist is your livelihood, art making is likely to be one part of your life rather than the center of it. Most of us have other obligations, to work, family, friends, self-care, or service to others. For us, there has to be a path down the middle, a path that respects that there are other things that fill our lives in addition to creativity.

The story of the historic Buddha is a good example for all of us on the path in between. When the prince Siddhartha Gautama, who was to become the Buddha, was born, seers predicted that he would either become a great king or save humanity. In response to this prediction, his father raised Siddhartha in a wealthy and pleasure-filled palace in order to shield him from any experience of human misery or suffering. He wanted to make sure that his son became a king rather than a savior.

Nonetheless, Siddhartha did witness several sights that changed the direction of his life: he saw a sick man, an old man, a corpse, and a wandering renunciate monk. These sights filled him with infinite sorrow for the suffering of old age, sickness, and death that humanity has to undergo, and he vowed to find a way to end human suffering. Inspired by the example of the renunciate monk, Siddhartha abandoned his indulgent way of life and dedicated himself to a life of extreme asceticism. This harsh practice, however, caused him to grow so thin that he could feel his hands if he placed one on the small of his back and the other on his stomach. In his weakened state, he happened to overhear a teacher saying that if the strings on a musical instrument are set too tight, then the instrument will not play harmoniously. If the strings are set too loose, the instrument will not produce music. Only the "middle way," not too tight and not too loose, will produce harmonious music.

This chance meeting was the turning point in Siddhartha's search. He realized that the way to reach his goal was not to live a completely worldly life, nor was it to live a life in complete denial of the physical body, but to follow the middle way of moderation. This approach is especially appropriate for "householders," ordinary people who wish to pursue a spiritual life without giving up their family and work obligations as a monk or full-time practitioner would do. We who are on the householder's path can try to find a balance, a middle path that offers us the pleasure of creativity in our lives along with regular spiritual practice. You don't have to set up a fully stocked studio and spend every waking moment to reap the benefits of the soul's palette. Be conscious of how the powers of imagination fit into the overall balance of your life and your needs for self-expression.

In the next chapter, you will learn how to set the stage for the soul's palette in your life and how to let go any inner voices that are holding you back from fully enjoying art's gifts.

THREE

Embracing Your Creative Birthright

*T*he famous art historian Ananda Coomaraswamy once noted that an artist is not a special kind of person but rather that every person is a special kind of artist.[1] Identifying your uniqueness as an artist and utilizing your natural ability to make images are the first steps to accessing your soul's palette. The activities in this chapter will help you begin to understand your uniqueness as an artist, rediscover your inner artistic source, and access your own creative capacity for personal healing. They will help you to dispel common myths about artistic creativity, remove barriers and obstacles to your creative wisdom, and learn to believe that you are an artist. By the end of this chapter you will have the inner resources to begin art making for personal expression.

To deepen your experience of rediscovery, this chapter also introduces transformational practices that will help you maintain your creativity and connection to the wisdom of the soul's palette. These practices are designed to help you get started in reclaiming your visual vocabulary and imagination.

YOUR PERSONAL ART MYTHOLOGY

From the first art class I taught in a public high school through my current work as an art therapist, I have come to realize that everyone has what I call a "personal art mythology." That is, each of us has developed a unique set of beliefs about what art is and what the words *painting* and *drawing* mean. The word *art* conjures up many definitions, memories, and images. For many, art is simply one of the great paintings or sculptures of history. For others, it may be street graffiti or a beautifully designed interior. For some, it is what puts them in touch with the sacred or sublime, whether it be an ancient temple or a magnificent landscape. For centuries, scholars, art historians, and critics have argued about what makes great art, and personal styles, tastes, and politics have dictated which works hang in an exhibition or museum. We have all been influenced in some way by these standards, rules, and authorities.

We may also have more personal reactions as a result of life experiences and a set of beliefs that have influenced how we see art, how it is created, and even who creates it. Family, friends, and our own inner voices can mold our perceptions, causing us to think that art is an activity only for the very talented or those with special skills. We may believe that there is a certain way of making images that is acceptable or that indicates a gift for creativity. You may have encountered powerful cultural taboos and events that stopped you from developing your creative source. You may also have been encouraged to make art, but in a way that discouraged your true voice and vision. All these influences, definitions, and beliefs affect how you feel about the creative source within.

Matisse once said, "It has bothered me all my life that I do not paint like everybody else." For many of us, this is exactly the thought that keeps us from tapping our creative source. Luckily, any loss of your artist self is not permanent; in fact, once you have revisited your imagination, you can easily reclaim it.

RECLAIMING WHAT WAS LOST

Losing touch with artistic imagination is, to some extent, part of growing up. While art, play, and creativity are central to early childhood, as we get older they often take a backseat to reading, writing, and mathematics. Imagination, drawing, painting, and making things with one's hands become less important than other ways of communicating.

Our own inner voices may stop us from artistic expression. For example, as teenagers we may be very intrigued with making drawings that look real but may not have the skill to create photographically realistic images. In frustration, many of us give up art altogether. As a result, most of us surrender what was once a natural activity of childhood and, as adults, feel that we cannot make art, cannot draw, and are not creative. We may even apologize for our lack of talent.

Artist Howard Ikemoto relates the following story: "When my daughter was about seven years old, she asked me one day what I did at work. I told her I worked at the college, that my job was to teach people how to draw. She stared back at me, incredulous, and said, 'You mean they forget?'"[2] If you are in a room filled with preschoolers and ask, "Who knows how to draw?" all the children will raise their hands. If you venture into a college classroom and ask the same question, it is likely that not a single hand will be raised. Somewhere between childhood and adulthood we often lose our connection with imagination and creative expression.

Most of us need help getting back the artist that was lost in childhood. Sometimes this involves remembering that creative spark each of us experienced as a child. For some of us, it involves recalling what events caused us to lose that spark and believe that creativity was not for us. When faced with the prospect of drawing or painting, we may remember a memory of childhood art making, usually a traumatic one that caused us to be fearful of art making later as adults. We may even experience with sadness how difficult it is to remember those moments in childhood when we painted or handled clay with great abandon and confidence in our creative spirit.

Luckily, we have often had positive experiences, too. Some of us remember a paint-by-number set, a piece of needlework or handicraft taught to us, or an art project in school that earned an A. Perhaps you remember a supportive parent, grandparent, or teacher who encouraged and nurtured your creative talents, or remember a time when you made a special drawing or object that gave you pride and satisfaction in your accomplishment. You may remember coloring, cutting, and pasting colored paper as a young child, and may have looked forward to art class each week or worked with an art teacher who came to visit your school on occasion. Unfortunately, the negative experiences are generally easier to remember. Some of these memories may prevent us from engaging in art making or other creative endeavors as adults, fearing that we will fail or that we are not truly artists.

I have heard countless stories from friends, clients, and colleagues recalling the exact moment when they decided that they could not paint or draw and had no artistic talent. They may also recount frustrations with the process of art making, saying, "I can't make it look real," or "I am not talented in art." At times these memories are so traumatizing that art making is forever banished as a possible creative outlet. In Antoine de Saint-Exupéry's famous tale *The Little Prince*, the narrator describes such a memory. He explains that as a child he once drew a picture of a snake that had swallowed an elephant. To his dismay, the adults looked at his picture and identified it as a hat. When he tried to show them that this was indeed a drawing of a snake with an elephant inside it, they continued to discount his description, misunderstanding the meaning of his picture. Sadly, he decided that he never wanted to draw again after that experience. I think the incident that Saint-Exupéry describes is common and often unfortunately causes both children and adults to put down their pencils and paintbrushes for good.

Because you may have stopped expressing yourself through art for many different reasons, childhood memories of art making can start to tell you where your soul's palette was lost and where to find it again. Pablo Picasso said, "Every child is born an artist." The problem is how to remain an artist once one grows up. A look back at what happened to the young artist you once were can renew your sense of self-exploration and restore authentic expression. Sometimes there is a lingering memory of a particular person who ridiculed your art, misunderstood what you were trying to communicate, or gave you a poor grade in an art class. Taking a mental inventory of memories, events, experiences, and attitudes about art that you developed during childhood is often helpful.

YOUR PERSONAL HISTORY AS AN ARTIST

An important first step in reclaiming your soul's palette includes revisiting your beliefs and remembering your personal history as an artist. Your childhood memories of art are sources of imagination, artistic creativity, and inner wisdom. When I begin work with people who may have been out of touch with art making for a long time, I often ask them to think about the places, events, and experiences that influenced their inner artist. By answering these questions you will begin to develop a sense of how images have influenced the course of your life. You will also begin to unlock the doors to your artistic imagination, intuition, and creative wisdom.

◆ What kind of art did you experience when you were growing up? Did it involve drawing and coloring? Crafts? Learning handiwork from a relative? Museum or gallery trips? Looking at paintings on the living room wall in your family's home? How did your family define art?

◆ What were the first art images that you were exposed to and that attracted or inspired you as a child? Book covers? Cartoons? *Life* magazine? Your cereal bowl? Your grandmother's pottery? A painting in a friend's home? Collect some of these types of images in the form of photographs or magazine clippings to make a collage or make simple sketches of them with color and lines.

◆ Did you have a favorite creative activity when you were young? Coloring books, paint-by-number, embroidery, knitting, building things? What do you remember about this activity?

◆ Did you ever have a negative experience with art when you were a child? For example, were you told that you were not artistic, that your older sibling was the artist in the family, or that your art expressions were not good enough?

◆ When you were a child, can you remember how you drew the sun, your house, a tree, a flower, your pet, and yourself? Try a simple sketch of these images, drawing like a five-year-old.

◆ Where did you do your drawings? In the kitchen? On the living room floor? In your bedroom? Were you alone, or were others present?

◆ What important or secret object or treasure did you hide under your pillow or bed? What made it special? Did it have any magical powers or meaning? Do you still have this object, or wish to have it?

◆ What in nature visually inspired or frightened you? Animals, the forest, the ocean, storms, wind? What did you imagine that you saw or heard in the dark or during a thunderstorm?

◆ What fairy tale, story, or film affected you when you were a young child? Is it still important now? Can you relate its characters and symbols to your life as an adult? Locate a storybook or tape about this tale and revisit it.

As a child you may have put away bit by bit the excitement of your imagination and your creative source, losing contact with the soul's palette. Use these questions to reacquaint yourself with visual details or memories of your childhood artist. The images you retrieve will help you to unlock some of your intuitive power and rediscover the artistic inspiration you have always had.

MAKING ART WITH AUTHENTICITY

For many of us, the first experiences making art took place with a parent or caretaker who cared deeply about us and brought art into our lives to nurture and enrich us. My earliest art making started with my mother, who encouraged me in every way she could. She taught me to embroider, bought me paint sets and craft kits, and took me to local art shows. She carefully saved many of my early paintings and poems in her hope chest and praised me for my skills and talent. At a very early age I felt very special about creativity and began to feel like a real artist.

At the same time, these first art experiences also complicated my perceptions of who I was really making art for and why I was creating it. While my mother truly wanted me to develop my imagination and creativity, these first art experiences had a powerful influence on the way I made art for many years. I became involved in producing images to please my mother and my family rather than developing an authentic way of self-expression. While making art for others is not always a bad thing, if we have failed to honor our true creative voice, it may take years to rediscover and recover.

Creating for people other than myself was reinforced in my first years in grade school. I vividly remember learning how to cut and paste paper onto a background to make what was probably my first collage in first grade. I recall my excitement handling the colorful papers, learning to use a scissors, and discovering all the forms I could create. I also remember the teacher directing me to look at her example on the front wall of the classroom, showing me what she intended for me to copy. That impressed me profoundly, so much so that I began earnestly to replicate drawings and images that the teacher presented each week. One time I drew a rose exactly according to her pattern, and the teacher lavished praise on me for my accuracy.

Truly, at that point, all my art making was a reflection of the visions of others. While I was delighting their souls with all my artwork, my own soul remained unnourished by art for many years. I had a really great-looking facade as someone who was talented at art, but inside there was something missing. I was busy making images for others, but I was not making art for myself. This is a familiar scenario for many of us during childhood, a loss of authentic expression that we often carry into adulthood.

During the fall of my eleventh year, I had the good fortune to be in a sixth-grade class with a teacher who recognized the value of self-expression. When I finished my reading or math, he would give me a box of art materials—paints, pencils, colored chalks, wrapping paper, and gold foils. He asked me if I would like to decorate the classroom doors or create a mural on the large bulletin board in the corridor. In the beginning, my own vision for making art was so undernourished that I had a terrible time thinking of images on my own. To help me recapture my imagination, he would give me a theme, like "birds of South America" or "life on another planet," and that would be my starting point for creating.

Rather than instructing me to reproduce the images he valued, my teacher facilitated my creative vision. My authenticity was accepted and my personal imagery nurtured; suddenly my whole world changed. I was a good student in grade school, but I usually lacked confidence in my abilities and ideas. Often I would have the right answer to a math problem or science question, but my lack of belief in myself prevented me from communicating. Now I was no longer so shy, and to my parents' amazement, I began to talk in class. I suddenly let go of all my fears, something totally out of character for me until then. I think what happened was simple—I found my artist's soul for the very first time, and my whole being was rejoicing in it. My newly discovered passion of using my imagination often brought me to school a half hour early to work on a picture, and I stayed late in the afternoon to add touches to a display or bulletin board. It carried me through all parts of the day and enlivened everything in my world and within me.

That year redefined for me what it meant to be an artist and to express oneself fully, freely, and authentically. I measured all future experiences with art making by the experience my sixth-grade teacher gave me. Later, when I was a student at the School of the Museum of Fine Arts in Boston, I quickly drifted away from studio classes that disrespected the internal sense of artist that I had developed. One instructor had us carefully draw human anatomy from a model for several hours, only to force us to wad up our labored creations and toss them in basketball fashion into a large trash can at the end of class. Another insisted that we paint huge abstract canvases as was the fashion at the time. In addition to my lack of interest in making monumental abstract paintings, I had the added struggle of getting six-foot-square canvases onto Boston subway cars. I quickly realized that I was back to making art for somebody else rather than me. While I continued to try to glean what I needed to know as an artist and obtain my degree, I knew deep inside that this was not the path I wanted to travel after I completed my degree.

Many years later, I faced an even greater struggle to retain my artist's soul and my authentic voice when I was a professor in an art department at a major university. Now that I look back, I see how inhibiting that environment was to true self-expression. A certain style of making art was subtly enforced, and the goal was to exhibit and sell one's work commercially. I listened to countless students behind closed doors of my office confide to me how they felt pressured to conform in order to please an instructor, get a good grade, or finish their degree. Surprisingly, the art historians were the worst, passing critical judgment on what art should be, while at the same time not engaging in artistic expression themselves. I found myself making less art during those years than at any other time of my life, my creative spirit literally drying up inside me.

I could easily have been another art school casualty—those who never recover from having their soul's expressions stifled by the more insensitive experiences of art education. And I could have felt that I was a failure, finding it impossible to remain on a university faculty, something many artists only dream of achieving. The soul's palette exists not to mold us into the images that others value but to celebrate the imagination that is unique to ourselves. Only through experiencing and expressing that uniqueness is the power of art as a source of well-being and soulful awakening tapped.

Over the years I developed and experimented with the activities and practices in this book, I had to reframe and reconstruct much of what I was taught in art school. For those who have not had formal art instruction, other voices may be calling. You may hear a small voice saying, "Don't waste materials making something stupid-looking," or "You can't draw or paint, you don't have any talent." Many people report thinking, "Making art is frivolous; there are many more important things to do with my time."

To engage your soul's palette, allow yourself to reshape your beliefs about artistic expression. First, don't worry about technical skills; there will be no grades and no judgments about whether or not your drawings or paintings are good enough. This time you do not have to color within the lines. Using the creative activities and the transformational practices in this book does not require you to have years of training in art or advanced skill. Also, remember when first starting out that your immediate goal is not to produce a beautiful painting or sculpture but to express yourself, take pleasure in the artistic process, and see what emerges. Try to let go of worries about the quality of your work and simply enjoy the process of creating.

KNOW YOUR INNER AND OUTER CRITICS

Although making art and tapping one's creative source can be therapeutic, pleasurable, or inspirational, it is not unusual to wonder whether
the painting or drawing one has made is good. We all have many internal voices that form judgments about our creative work, particularly in art making, where a tangible product remains. Part of the joy
in making art is producing something that visually pleases you and
inspires you to use your creative source even more.

Reshaping your art mythology involves looking at the art critics
in our lives and within ourselves. Not all critics are necessarily bad; in
fact, some can actually help artistic expression. Critics, whether they
are actual people or internal voices, make us think, help us make ad-
justments, and surprise us when we get too complacent. The message
they carry, when given in an atmosphere of support, sparks our imagination, nurtures self-expression, and stokes the creative fire. Critics
can get in the way, however, when they pass judgment without supporting the creative process and impose rules and standards that do
not honor the image or its creator.

The following creative activities may help you explore your inner
and outer critics:

◆ If you find yourself repeatedly asking yourself whether your work
is good or correct, spend some time exploring where this is coming
from. Write down what your inner voices say and think about whether
those voices are coming from you or from parents, partners, teachers,
bosses, or others.

◆ Create a simple mask to identify the inner and outer art critic and
other internal censors. Use collage materials (magazine images of people and printed statements are particularly good), scissors, glue, and
felt marking pens, and a paper plate as a template for a face. Cut the
plate to reflect the shape of a face and, if you wish, cut out holes for
eyes, nose, and mouth. On one side of the mask, glue pictures and
words that represent the outer critic—a teacher, boss, parent, or other
authority who criticized your creative abilities. On the other side,
arrange images and words that come from the critic within you.

◆ How would your mask image look if the inner critic within was actually your companion on the journey, someone who is always with you to guide you rather than shame you? Sometimes our own critical voice (as opposed to someone else's) can help us to make decisions to use a little more blue paint, erase a line, or simply start all over again. Recognizing that inner voice as a guide or reframing it as a confidant can be helpful on the path to opening and restoring the soul's palette. Try making a mask of your companion critic to serve as a guide and a mentor for your creative expression.

TRY NOT-KNOWING

Traditional Eastern philosophies have a great deal to teach us about finding and cherishing our natural creative abilities. Zen master Seung Sahn and Pema Chödrön, a leading voice in the American tradition of Tibetan Buddhism, remind us about "don't-think mind," the place where valuable teachings arise, wiser than anything we learn in the world. The ancient Taoist master Lao-tzu taught, "Practice not-doing and everything will fall into place." One of the things that artistic creativity has to teach us is to let go and go with what emerges in our more innocent moments of awareness. No matter how many times we sit down with pencils and paper or a lump of clay, we need to continually relearn how to create with a beginner's innocence, curiosity, and exploration.

Try to begin with simple acceptance of your imagination and creativity. Milton Erickson, one of the world's most renowned hypnotherapists, would consciously go into trances of not-knowing before working with a patient. He believed that creative forgetting allows people to discover new potentials within themselves. When you stop knowing, a space naturally opens for new information to come in. In artistic expression you often have to be open to unlearning what you already believe and make room for knowing in a new way. The mode of not-knowing, Erickson observed, permits images within you to come forth and new ways of experiencing your creative source to emerge.

In his writings about creativity, art therapist Shaun McNiff has pointed out, time after time, that real transformation occurs when one simply "trusts the process." When one lets oneself enter the river and goes with the flow, great changes occur and wonderful things happen. Mysteriously, answers emerge and problems begin to resolve. The path of art making asks you to act on faith. In taking a stance of not-knowing, you trust the process, accept that what you are creating is right for you in the moment, and have faith that the universe supports your creative source.

Think of not-knowing as what Steve Nachmanovitch, author of *Free Play: Improvisation in Art and Life*, calls "disappearing." In order for art to appear, we often have to disappear, allowing our minds and senses to become quiet for the moment. Fully involving yourself in creativity in this way will help you to let go of worrying about what your images look like and allow you to enjoy the process of creating them. In other words, try not to become distracted with yourself or by yourself. Disappear, find that quiet place inside, and make room for your creativity to emerge.

These creative activities can help you understand the concept of not-knowing:

◆ Take some time to go to a place in nature that you enjoy, or a museum, gallery, or sculpture garden—someplace where there are images to delight and stimulate your senses. When you arrive, just wander around without anything on your mind. Observe what is there— trees, a fountain, flowers, paintings, sculptures—and let your intuition guide you as to what to do next. Look at objects and images you are attracted to, but try not to analyze what you see. Experiment with not-knowing, and look at objects and images as if you were seeing them for the first time, simply experiencing them.

You can use this as a one-time activity, but experiment with this practice on a regular basis. You will find that it is naturally calming and will help you to approach artistic expression with a sense of curiosity as well as to develop your skills in tapping into don't-know mind.

◆ While your own art making is important, try also looking for don't-know mind in others. One of the best ways to do this is to watch a group of young children create, scribble, draw, paint, play-act, or dance. They engage in don't-know mind through creative expression without rules. Watch them with a beginner's eye and feel the joy and inhibition of their artistic expression.

PAY ATTENTION TO YOUR SYMBOLS

You can begin to reshape your inner creative source through paying attention to how you respond to images that you see around you. Each of us consciously or unconsciously chooses to have visual symbols—images and objects—in our environments. We all are drawn to certain colors, shapes, forms, patterns, and textures in our environment or may consciously place them around us in decorating our home or choosing outfits to wear. We also keep pictures, prints, photographs, cards, or objects in our homes or offices, images and items that have importance to us, remind us of a person, memory, or event, or simply give us pleasure when looking a them. These visual symbols tell a lot about what and how we value images.

For example, I keep the following visual symbols close by in my office space: a basket of hand-dyed yarns I collected in California; photos of family, friends, the family cats, and a memorable trip to China; a large Monet print my husband purchased at a museum; books on Georgia O'Keeffe's paintings and the Mexican celebration of the Day of the Dead; assorted plastic animals and dinosaurs that sit on my printer; a photo of a large rock I took on the Atlantic coast; a Magritte art print; and a small pile of sand dollars I picked up on the coast of Oregon. These are visual images that give me pleasure, help me to recall gratifying and important events, and are a source and inspiration for artistic expression. When I am going through a mental block in writing, I often leaf through the book of O'Keeffe paintings to relax my mind, enjoy the textures of natural objects on display, or rearrange and play with the animals on my printer to escape from my work for a few minutes.

Take some time to pay attention to the visual symbols you encounter, and think about your answers to the following questions:

◆ What colors and textures do you like to have in your environment?

◆ What images are significant in your home?

◆ Do you keep photos of family and friends in your office or family room?

◆ Do you hang prints or calendars with special images on your walls? Are they pictures of nature, animals, or a certain artist's paintings you enjoy?

◆ What objects do you like to have around you?

◆ Pick a room at home in which you keep the most personal images and objects. Take some time to write down a few phrases about each image or object. Try to note why you like each particular image: for example, you like the color or shape, or the image makes you feel happy or peaceful, or it reminds you of a particular experience or event.

By identifying and learning what images and objects are meaningful to you, you begin to identify what visual symbols you value. We generally collect and keep symbols around us that are meaningful. The composition and arrangement of these symbols, whether consciously or unconsciously planned, is an environmental collage that says a lot about what you value, what images you appreciate, and what images bring you joy, pleasure, and inspiration. These symbols not only tell you about your visual preferences but can also serve as a source of inspiration for your imagination and creative process.

HONOR YOUR CREATIVE AUTHORITY

The thirteenth-century Chinese sage Wu-men said, "The Great Way has no gate. There are a thousand paths to it." Although you may believe that there is only one right way to engage your artistic expression, in fact there are a thousand paths springing from your imagination and your ability to create images for growth, reparation, and transformation—and you have a unique ability and authority to use these inner resources. Honor this creative authority in yourself. Be generous to yourself and find your own path of art and imagination that gives you pleasure, inspiration, and a sense of well-being.

Although I have spent much of my adult life guiding others in finding their artistic creativity, I don't think of myself as an expert about what is right for others. I know a lot about how art has touched me and why art has become a wellness practice in my own life. I have also been fortunate and humbled to witness many individuals' experiences of art making and personal transformation. Despite this background, I am not an authority on the process of art making for others. Honoring your own creative authority is the most important element in calling forth your soul's palette and is a powerful factor in art's capacity to renew and restore. In the next chapter you will learn how to help this creative authority thrive through knowing materials and creating a space for your soul's palette to flourish.

Knowing Materials and Creating Space

rt making is a hands-on activity, involving constructing, arranging, mixing, touching, molding, gluing, drawing, stapling, painting, and forming. But without materials, there is no art. This chapter gives you practical information on the materials of drawing, painting, sculpting, and collage—and how, why, and when to use these materials to stimulate your creative journey. You will learn that each art medium has a different personality and mission, and how you can use these to inspire your creative work.

In this chapter you will also learn how to create a studio as a sanctuary to nourish your creative source. You will discover how to make your own artist's studio, which can be a part of your kitchen or family room, the outdoors, a space at your desk at work, a sketchbook, or even a moment in time. Knowing materials and creating space will give your soul's palette the necessary tools to flourish and will fuel your intention to make artistic creativity a regular part of your life.

MATERIALS

I like art materials almost as much as I like art making itself. I like to savor art material catalogues and wander in art stores wherever and whenever I can. There is something uplifting about seeing all the different brushes, papers, pastels, and paints, smelling the scents, and touching boxes and sketchpads that fills me with anticipation and starts my mind imagining new projects.

I respect materials as friends, and, just like friends, each one has a different personality. Some are colorful and bold, others are sensual and long to be touched, some are graceful and quiet, and many are inviting and energizing. You can use these personalities to enhance your work with art as a wellness practice. As you read about each material and its personality, consider which one resonates with you right now.

I believe that each material has a different mission for creative expression. That is, each lends itself to communicating feelings, telling stories, or reconstructing and reframing ideas—or a combination of some or all of the above. In the sections that follow, you will see how drawing, painting, clay sculpture, and collage have unique missions that employ the many potentials of the soul's palette to express, reflect, and resolve.

Drawing Materials

Everybody knows how to draw. We doodle while on the phone, create diagrams of the layout of a room or vegetable garden, or sketch projects we want to undertake or things we plan to make. As children, we use drawing as a form of language to communicate events and experiences for which we do not yet have words. We draw to express what we see and what we imagine.

Drawings use line as their basic element. Lines define shapes, create boundaries, lead the eye, express rhythm, and take us from one place to another. There is not a right way or wrong way to use a line, nor is there a wrong way to draw.

Although you can certainly express your feelings through lines, forms, and colors, drawing's special mission as a form of self-expression is narration. It is a way to tell stories, to talk and communicate through visual means. If hand-drawn lines were the only symbols you could use to communicate with, you would still have an endless source of symbols to say whatever you wanted to.

You can make lines and drawings with just about anything—your finger dipped in paint, a twig in the sand, or a ballpoint pen on a notepad. Don't be limited by the notion that all drawings are made on paper. You can draw lines in space with your hands, feet, and body without ever making a mark on a surface. However, there are some traditional drawing materials to get acquainted with—pencils, charcoal, ink, crayons, pens, and pastels.

Pencils. When I was a first-year art student, I had at least fifty pencils. They were mostly graphite—the black mineral that, mixed with clay, forms the core of what we often refer to as "lead" pencils that come in various degrees of hardness and softness measured in numbers. The familiar #2 pencil is usually used for writing, while softer pencils offer different effects for drawing. I preferred the ones that made the darkest and most emphatic marks on paper. Every time I visited an art store, it was exciting to buy a few more pencils even if I didn't need them. I liked to always have some new ones handy to start a drawing series or just to display on my work table in a large glass jar.

Pencils are the traditional foundation of drawing. They are used to make art, but are also related to problem-solving activities in image making. You might use them to sketch plans for future works or diagrams, or to solve a problem visually. Because you can erase most pencil lines, the material is very forgiving and lets you keep your options open. You can also change pencil lines with something as simple as your finger or a soft cloth, blurring the edges and blending marks together.

There are also colored pencils in a rich variety of hues and intensities. I like to use colored pencils to draw images when I feel the need to slow down. They force you to focus on working within small spaces and invite you to shade, layer colors, and add details to images.

Ink. Ink is often spontaneous and dramatic as a drawing material. The lines that can be made with black ink on paper are like no others made with pencil or charcoal. They are definite, often bold, and generally flowing and organic. They can also be precise and controlled, depending on how ink is applied to a surface.

Pen and ink is often used to achieve tight, fine lines and detailed shading by layering lines one upon the other. There are quill pens that you can dip into ink to make lines, and there are mechanical pens that are for the same purpose. I recommend staying with the old-fashioned quill type, because mechanical pens, despite advances in technology, tend to clog and require a lot of attention to keep them clean and working. Pen and ink has sort of an uptight personality, so I enjoy it when I want to work small, include lots of details, and feel a bit obsessive.

A more expressive way of working with ink is with a brush. Any good brush can be used, but traditionally sumi brushes are preferred. These are usually handmade in Asia and are soft, absorbent, natural-hair brushes with bamboo handles used in traditional Japanese black ink painting (*sumi-e*) and calligraphy. They can also be used to draw with ink or with watercolors and other types of paints. Sumi ink traditionally comes in a stick that you grind in water, but you can also buy it by the bottle. There is a rich history and ritual to sumi painting; using these materials in your own way evokes some of that history while allowing you to enjoy the spontaneity of drawing with these materials.

Any kind of black ink can be thinned with water to create gray tones. There also are a wide variety of colored and metallic inks available, generally through art supply stores.

Oil pastels. Oil pastels, sold under brand names such as Cray-Pas, are soft, greasy drawing sticks that come in a variety of colors, from light pastel shades to intense, brilliant colors. If you are just starting out, this is one of the easiest materials to work with. Oil pastels blend freely and are a good choice for most drawing activities. Because they are vivid in color, it is hard to be timid with them. The marks that are made with oil pastels are bold and permanent, so if you are feeling tentative and dainty, they may not be the material for you.

Most oil pastels can be thinned with a little turpentine on a soft cloth or brush to blur the edges or blend colors; if you decide to do this, just be sure to work in a well-ventilated area or open a window. Some oil pastels are actually water-soluble, meaning you can use a little water on your fingertip or a brush to mix and blend colors in your drawings.

Crayons. Crayons are somewhat like oil pastels and have a symbolic association to childhood for most people. For many of us, they were the first materials we used in visual expression, usually to create scribbles for a watchful parent. You may still enjoy using crayons to draw;

the joy of having and handling a new box of crayons may be, in itself, your source of creative inspiration.

One drawback of crayons is that they do not have the range of color and possibilities for mixing that oil pastels offer. I suggest you try a set of adult crayons from an art supply store. If you can spend a bit more, buy a set of Caran D'Ache water-soluble crayons. They are a kind of hybrid between oil pastels and crayons and come in deep, brilliant colors. They are much more sensually satisfying than the crayons that came in the green and yellow box.

Chalk pastels. Chalk pastels are a hands-on material that forces you to get your fingers dirty. You can't get caught in details when using these pastels because they are powdery and somewhat like blackboard chalk. You can blend them and use them to create soft lines and edges. Their dreamy quality is like no other, and you will find yourself having to forgive them because they smear easily once applied to a surface. Be careful to protect anything in your space that you do not want covered with colored chalk dust. Use a spray fixative to protect your work from smudging. Ordinary hairspray will work, or you can purchase an artist's fixative at a supply store; be sure to have adequate ventilation when spraying.

Felt pens. If you like vibrant colors and bold lines, felt-tip marking pens are easy to use and readily available. Because they are permanent, I like to use them when I feel emphatic or assertive. They come in a wide range of colors with fine or broad tips; be sure to try both types.

Drawing surfaces. Just about anything can be your surface for a drawing. Two of the most common are paper and paper-based board. The most popular is paper, which comes in smooth and rough varieties. For drawings with chalk pastels, for example, you will need a paper or surface with texture in order for it to hold the medium. There are many beautiful papers available, but any kind of paper can be your drawing surface. Consider the humble brown paper bag, interesting envelopes, legal pads, and even the backs of business cards.

"Board" commonly refers to illustration board, museum board, and even cardboard; various types of boards are available at art supply stores. Board is more durable than paper because it is thicker and more resistant to damage. If you have a chance, visit an art store and look over the various kinds of drawing board that are available.

Creative Activities: Drawing

To learn more about the personalities of drawing materials, try the following creative activities.

Self-stick notepad sketches. If you are just starting out, you may feel more comfortable with drawing on small surfaces. Try drawing with thin-tipped felt pens or even ballpoint pens on self-stick notes (such as Post-it brand notes) or small notepads. Start with simple scribbling and doodling and see what evolves. You may find if you keep an on-going Post-it note sketchbook that your initial scribbles start to find their own rhythms, movement, and forms. When young children draw, their first images are scribbles, chaotic mazes of lines that are spontaneous and unorganized. This chaos eventually becomes orderly, and shapes and form emerge from the lines. Your drawings will have the same natural tendency of art to find order.

Some of the most fun I have drawing on small surfaces is with a set of gel pens and black Post-it notes. Gel pens are like ballpoint pens except they come in very bright, intense colors and flow very smoothly onto paper and other surfaces. Drawing on a black background is a novel experience. Forms and images seem to pop out of the darkness, and you may find that you are more expressive on black paper than on white.

Nondominant-hand drawing. Letting your nondominant hand draw (as opposed to your dominant hand, the one you use for writing) is a great way to let go and let loose. Most of us cannot control our non-dominant hand, so expect your lines and forms to do as they wish rather than as you want. Try this activity with a large piece of drawing paper, and simply let your nondominant hand wander around the space, using a crayon, oil pastel, or chalk pastel. You can also experiment by drawing with both hands at once. Your hands may draw mirror images, or you may find yourself creating two completely different pictures.

"Kill the hand." Another way to approach drawing is expressed in the Zen saying "Kill the hand." In order to kill your hand's control over drawing, tie a small piece of cloth or chamois to the end of a stick about three feet long, dip it in ink, and draw on a large piece of paper tacked on a wall. Hold the stick at its end, not the center, otherwise you won't get the desired effect. Losing a little control of your hand in this way will free your lines and transfer a different kind of energy onto the paper.

Drawing the heart of the image. When I was in art school, drawing was usually taught in one of two ways. Sometimes I was instructed to draw what I saw—that is, to portray figures, objects, and nature in a representational, realistic way. At other times I was taught to be very design conscious and focus on composition, pattern, and style.

I think there is a more authentic way to draw than either of these approaches. It involves what you *sense* about images rather than what you see. Try drawing the heart of the image by using gesture as your approach. *Gesture* is another word for movement, and gesture drawing is another way of connecting to the essence of an image. If you are drawing from life, try looking at the object in front of you as if you were experiencing its energy or life force. If you are drawing from your imagination, go with the emotion of that image and use your pencil or pastel to create gestural movements on the drawing surface. See if you can connect with the whole object rather than any one detail.

Think of drawing as a way to recognize the heart of the object or inner image you want to express. In approaching drawing in this way, you will inevitably touch your own core—your heart and spirit—and express the language of your own feelings.

Dance your drawing. If you are feeling really daring or just want to experience cutting loose, try using body movement as a source for drawing. Get a large piece of butcher or craft paper, at least three feet wide and six feet long or more. Tape it to the wall either horizontally or vertically. Put on some music that suits your mood, take oil or chalk pastel in hand, and move your hands and body to the music. Transfer some of those movements to the paper with bold lines and

strokes, changing colors as it feels appropriate. The lines
may become the end point of your drawing, or you may us
a starting point for additional embellishment and to encou
ages to emerge from the patterns.

Just experiment. Try doodling on different size papers and different
surfaces. See how many different kinds of lines you can make with a
ballpoint pen on a page from a yellow legal pad, or try using oil pastels on a piece of wax paper. How many surfaces can become places
where you can make lines, shapes, and images? Notice what sizes and
textures are comfortable for your expression.

Painting Materials

Like drawing, painting can communicate a story, but its true mission
is to tap and express feelings. Paint is sensuous, fluid, and sometimes
difficult to control. Each time you pick up a brush to paint, there is a
potential to express something gentle or bold or spectacular. Paint
has a unique personality: it can be stimulating because of the color
and brushstrokes, and at the same time hypnotic and almost sedating
because of its fluidity.

Painting is a metaphor for many things. It has taught me on numerous occasions that not everything in life can be planned and that
my expectations are often quite different from what actually happens. Because it is so fluid and uncontrollable, paint helps me to surrender the need to control and teaches me literally to go with the
flow. It also has taught me patience and flexibility, especially when I
get too comfortable and confident in my artistic expression. Paint
seems to have a mind of its own at times, and I am continually learning how to work in tandem with it, rather than struggling to always
make it do what I want in the moment.

There are several kinds of paints that are easy to use for beginners.

Tempera. Tempera paint comes in liquid form in bottles and in a variety of vibrant colors. It is nontoxic and water-soluble, cleans up easily, and dries quickly. Start with at least white, black, red, yellow,
blue, and brown; if you like bright colors, add to that list magenta,

orange, turquoise, green, and purple. You may want to have a little extra white, yellow, and red on hand to mix with other colors.

Watercolors. Watercolor invites experimenting, imagination, and play. Watch a group of preschoolers with their first set of tray watercolors and you will witness the wonder of this painting material. Young children are fascinated not only by the marks they can make putting brush to color and then to paper but also by watching the colors float and whirl in a clear glass of water.

Watercolors teach you about transparency, spontaneity, and trusting the process. They also are a metaphor for permanence, because once you commit them to paper, you cannot go back and change things. Watercolors teach me to accept the way my actions turn out and to leave things alone rather than try to rework them. One of my painting teachers once said, "It takes two people to make a watercolor—one to paint it and the other to stop him before he ruins it."

If your studio space is small or you like to work with compact materials, tube watercolors are a good choice. The concentrated pigment goes a long way. Start with the same palette of colors as tempera.

Acrylics. Acrylics are another good choice because they are convenient and versatile. They come in tubes, and you can start with the same color palette as tempera. They were once viewed as poor substitutes for the more traditional oil paints but now are popular because they are easy to use and clean up with water.

Acrylic is not quite as fluid as tempera paints, but there are artist's mediums that you can mix with them to thin them and retard their drying time. I like acrylics because, like watercolors, they are direct and give immediate results. They are also forgiving; once the painting is dry, you can paint over sections of your image, so there is always an opportunity to recover from any mistakes. Acrylics let you experiment in a number of ways: you can use them on just about any surface, mix them with sand for texture, and make marks in wet paint to create lines and patterns.

Painting surfaces. Paper and canvas are two traditional surfaces for painting. You can paint directly on paper, or you can prepare the surface with a substance known as gesso. Gesso comes in white and black, helps makes a surface impervious to liquid, and will strengthen paper to take large amounts of paint. Canvas, the generally accepted surface for painting with acrylics and oils, is often primed with gesso. You can paint on unprimed canvas; you might find yourself enjoying the way the surface absorbs the paint and the way the canvas gives under the pressure of your brush.

Watercolor is best used on special paper for that purpose. There are smooth, rough, and highly textured or toothy papers on which to apply watercolor. Buy the best grade you can afford, because it often makes a difference in the intensity of colors in your paintings.

Think of nontraditional surfaces for your creative expression. Try cardboard, newspaper, or pages from a discarded book or magazine as your surface. You can use any of these surfaces as they are or prepare them with a coat of acrylic paint or gesso.

Creative Activities: Painting

Don't-think mind. Painting is a perfect creative activity through which to practice "don't-think mind." Start with several large sheets of heavy paper or cardboard; use inexpensive surfaces so that you won't worry about making mistakes. Just keep painting, stay fully aware of what you are doing, but try to stay in don't-think mind. If you think too much about it, you become overly cautious; that is not the way of paint.

If you feel like working on a smaller format, buy a set of blank watercolor postcards at an art supply store or cut watercolor paper into five-by-seven-inch pieces. Let loose don't-think mind and paint with abandon on the cards using watercolor, tempera, or acrylics. Use a brush or sponge, fingerpaint, or dip your cards directly into the paint. If you like very small surfaces, try using blank business cards and use a small brush and washes of color.

Taking a don't-think mind approach to painting can be a transformational practice, one worth repeating because it taps spontaneous imagery (see more about this in chapter 5). It helps you to relax with the process and establishes an environment of trust within yourself to allow your own images to unfold.

Make a bad painting. A Zen proverb says: When you try to stay on the surface of the water, you sink, but when you try to sink, you float. Like not-knowing, sometimes doing the opposite of what your mind is telling you to do brings about what you really want. Try painting a series of ugly pictures or use colors that you don't like or that your mind tells you don't complement each other.

You can adapt any of the drawing activities in the previous section by substituting paint. Try killing the hand, using your nondominant hand, painting the heart of the image, or dancing your painting. The goal is to affirm your trust in the process, in letting materials lead the way from your creative source.

Collage

I have an artist friend who uses only collage to create art. She loves the simplicity of cutting and arranging sections of photos and magazines to make new images. Basically, collage involves only three actions: tearing or cutting, composing, and adhering the composition to a surface with glue. Most of us have made a collage at one time or other during our lives, usually as children with colored construction paper and white school glue or sticky paste.

I like collage when I want to have a lot of choices of images and textures, need to feel some control, and want the option of changing my mind. Collage is a very forgiving media in that it does not demand a commitment right away like a brushstroke across a canvas. Until you glue down the collage, you have the possibility of changing the composition, moving pieces around, and experimenting with as many arrangements as necessary.

Collage's mission is to give a second life to papers, objects, and symbols. It is a way to create order from chaos and to birth new images from old. While the process involves placing images together on a surface, it also evokes the layering of ideas, thoughts, and feelings. Collage can be a form of visual biography because it is often composed of personal images, photographs, or memorabilia. It is truly a transformative experience of taking what already exists and finding unexpected associations and meanings by creating a new context.

Creative Activities: Collage

Gathering, sorting, and storing. For me, the most pleasurable stage of collage making is collecting. Don't threaten to throw anything out when I am around your home or office—everything has potential for a collage, either today or in the future. Many artists enjoy the thrill of the hunt for exotic papers and objects at flea markets, swap meets, and the neighbors' trash containers on collection day. Finding and collecting collage materials involves all the emotions that keep us engaged in living each day—discovery, anticipation, hope, potentiality, and expectation.

The process of collecting collage materials has three stages: gathering, sorting, and storing. Gathering is simply collecting any and all papers, photographic images, fabrics, leaves, string, and objects that you intuitively feel attracted to or enjoy. Start with old magazines and begin to cut or tear out images that appeal to you. Travel magazines such as *National Geographic*, or home and garden, fashion, and health magazines are good starting points for photo images. Postcards, interesting greeting cards, snapshots, and junk mail are some other resources. Look for words, sentences, or sayings in cards and magazines that attract you; you may find these useful to add to your images. Go to the hardware store and take home paint chips of colors that you like. You may also want to add swatches of colors from envelopes or wrapping paper, foil, tissue paper, and ribbons as well as feathers, leaves, or other natural materials.

After gathering a fair amount of collage materials, you will want to sort and store your collection. This will help you find what you need later on for other activities in this book and for future collage making. Use envelopes and small boxes, or treat yourself to some of those colorful plastic containers and baskets you have always wanted. Make a collage box out of a large cardboard box, or purchase and decorate an inexpensive archive box (a cardboard box with a lid) from an office supply store. Place everything in this box, or organize the materials into separate units to place in it.

The collage box is really a long-term practice because, as you explore your inner artist, you will continue to add materials and images to this box. This box will hold your seeds for creative activities, so make it a habit to collect images and materials, use your imagination, and enjoy the process.

Recycling drawings and paintings. Over decades of making art, I have made a lot of pieces that I can live without. I have old sketches, some images that were never quite finished, and paintings that were experiments or downright mistakes. These are all compost for the collage box and possible reincarnations to a new life and another image. Next time, their karmic destinies may be better than the first time around.

Try cutting a drawing or painting you have made, but are not satisfied with, into small squares. Rearrange these into another image, playing with the pieces and eliminating those you don't like. Use dressmaker pins to keep the pieces in place until you find a composition that you like. You can also try cutting a large drawing or painting into strips and weaving them together as you would a mat. You may be surprised to find that your previous artworks take on a more satisfying form when you have the option to arrange them into a new image.

Clay Modeling

Clay's mission is to help us express the soul's palette in three dimensions and see things from all sides. It allows us to create from many different vantage points and is a very dynamic material that gets your hands dirty. There are basically three kinds of clay:

Potter's clay is made of earth and water and is nature's most abundant art supply. It is the material that is used to create ceramic pots and sculptures and is very inexpensive. This type of clay may not be suitable for your space, because it requires a kiln or oven to harden it and ventilation (dry clay creates considerable dust). However, because it is so economical, it is a wonderful clay to have on hand to create figures, forms, and objects.

Synthetic modeling material, such as Plasticine, Fimo, or Play-Doh, is a form of clay that is great for spaces where no kiln is available. It comes in a large range of colors, from bright reds and blues to pastels and natural tones. It can be molded, sculpted, rolled, coiled, and carved without the dust and dirt of natural clay. Plasticine hardens but never really completely dries; it can be reworked at a future time if you want to use it again for another project.

Self-hardening clay, sometimes called Mexican clay, is like potter's clay except it will harden without firing in a kiln. It can be decorated when dry with acrylic paints. There are also synthetic self-hardening clays sold under brand names such as Model Magic and Sculpey. They are easy to use, very pliable, dry relatively quickly, come in many colors, and can be painted. For making small objects, these are best choices to have on hand.

Make your own. Here is a recipe for an inedible dough for ornamental baking, easy to make at home.

Combine 4 cups unsifted all-purpose flour with 1 cup salt in a bowl, and stir in 1 ½ cups water, mixing thoroughly with hands. If dough is too stiff to handle, add more water, a little at a time. Remove dough from bowl and knead on a board for 4–6 minutes. Shape into desired ornaments or roll out and cut with cookie-cutters. You can also make your own cookie-cutter shapes by cutting them out of cardboard, placing the cardboard shapes onto the rolled-out dough, and then using the point of a knife to cut around the shapes. Holes may be poked through the "cookies" so that, after they are baked and painted, you can string a ribbon through for hanging.

Bake your objects or "cookies" on baking sheets in a preheated 350-degree oven for one hour or more, depending on size and thickness. Test for doneness with a toothpick in the thickest part of the piece. If it is still soft, bake a little longer. Lift from the cookie sheet with a spatula. Cool on racks. When completely cooled, paint or decorate. Spray with a clear fixative to prevent softening.

The dough must be used within four hours or it will be too dry. Do not double or halve the recipe.

Creative Activities: Clay

Don't-think clay. Whatever clay you decide to use, try using don't-think mind with a piece of clay the size of your fist. Close your eyes and just roll the clay round in one or both hands for a minute. Try different motions—pressing, stroking, pulling, flattening, molding. Keep your eyes closed and continue experimenting until you find a shape emerging from the clay. Try to continue forming the clay without judgment until you feel satisfied with the object.

Breathing the clay. Clay touches many of our senses—sight, touch, and even smell. Its sensory personality can help you to clear your mind, shift your consciousness, and induce relaxation. To experience these qualities of clay, quietly hold a fistful of potter's clay or soft Plasticine in your hands. Close your eyes and let your entire body relax; some soft instrumental music can help, or try progressively relaxing each part of your body until you feel a sensation of calm. Become aware of your breathing, and slowly begin to press both your thumbs into the center of the clay in rhythm with your breath. Observe your breath and physical sensations, allowing them to direct your fingers' movement into the clay.

The goal is to try to match your finger movements to your breath. Move slowly and purposefully, continuing to work with the clay for at least fifteen minutes or until your experience feels complete. As with don't-think mind, the point is to stay out of your head and keep your focus on your breath and body.

Just play. Clay's personality has the ability to bring out the child in you. Try calling forth your spirit of play when using this medium. Start with some children's clay from a toy or hobby store—either self-hardening or cans of modeling compound such as Play-Doh. Have on hand a rolling pin, some old combs, pencils, plastic utensils, cookie cutters, and natural objects. Roll the clay flat between two sheets of waxed paper with the rolling pin. Use cookie cutters to make shapes, and try embossing the clay pieces with pencils, the combs, utensils, or natural objects.

Play is a state of being that enables us to feel free to explore and express without inhibition or self-judgment and to think flexibly and innovatively. Use clay work as an opportunity to practice being in a state of play, to develop your artistic confidence, and to try new ideas. Let yourself go; clay is a naturally forgiving medium because, until it has dried, it can be reincarnated into endless forms, objects, and structures. See what you can learn from clay about your own abilities to adapt, experiment, problem-solve, and take risks.

Found Materials

Some of the most satisfying art I have made has been created with found materials or objects from nature. One year I made a beautiful set of ornaments for our Christmas tree out of old light bulbs from a discarded light fixture and colored paper varnished onto the surfaces. A pile of outdated computer CDs were also transformed by decorating them with beads and sequins and a bit of paint. Our tree that season had a high-tech and homemade charm.

It is fulfilling to use things we might normally throw away to create something new. Found materials challenge us to think beyond what art materials have to be. Using materials we don't normally think of as potential art is also a liberating experience that can loosen the creative source within to think beyond its boundaries. We often imagine that the most expensive art supplies are the best and will result in good art. Using recycled, found, or free materials gives us permission to see the world itself as a source of art and imagination.

Children have shown me that art can be made from anything. Many years ago I worked for social services evaluating children for placement in foster homes. Part of my job was to make home visits with a social worker to families. One day my coworker called to tell me we were going on an unusual home visit that day to see a family who lived in their car in a poor area of the city. He also cryptically added, "I think you are going to be really interested in the children. They are good candidates for your art therapy program."

When we arrived to meet the family, I fully understood his comment. The children had constructed a series of houses out of large cardboard boxes, loose bricks, and wood scraps. Each of the structures was elaborately decorated with paper, flowers, sticks, and found objects. The parents reported that although other children in the neighborhood frequently destroyed the structures, their children continued to rebuild and embellish their houses. It was obvious that the children wanted a real home to live in, rather than the family station wagon.

But it was also easy to see that they were deeply engaged in making something creative out of their existence without access to sophisticated artist materials and supplies.

Assemblage is a term used for three-dimensional collage or sculpture made of junk and scraps. The piece that the children created out of boxes and recycled items could be called a kind of assemblage. Assemblage is about problem solving, taking a variety of unrelated objects and using them in connection with one another to make a composition. It is an opportunity to use things that have one meaning and combine them with others to create something with a completely different meaning.

Consider everything you normally throw away as trash as possible starting points for art making. Look at egg cartons, bottles, light bulbs, tin cans, and containers as objects you can decorate and embellish. Think about materials used in construction and home improvement projects—wire, duct tape, nails, hinges, plastic pipes—as additional sources. Consider nature as a source of assemblage, and collect leaves and twigs from your yard or shells and wood from a beach. A master of nature assemblage, British sculptor Andy Goldsworthy uses only what he finds in nature to create his pieces—stones, twigs, even icicles. Try your own nature assemblages by making an arrangement of river rocks on your desk, or fill a series of containers with interesting branches or tall weeds. As suggested for collage, practice gathering, sorting, and storing natural materials for future projects.

A BASIC ART KIT

The following materials are helpful to have on hand for the activities and practices in this book:

- Several graphite pencils, both soft and hard
- A bottle of black ink (washable variety)
- A set of 24 color oil pastels
- A set of 24 color chalk pastels
- A set of 12 color felt pens

- Tempera paints or acrylics (white, black, red, yellow, blue, brown, and additional colors you like)
- A small set of tube watercolors
- A large sketchpad with good-quality white paper (18 x 24 inches)
- At least five brushes of various sizes (buy the best quality you can afford)
- Collage and assemblage materials
- Scissors
- Glue sticks or white glue
- Self-hardening clay

STUDIOS: THE GIFT OF SANCTUARY

I love to walk into a space where art is being made. It can be an artist's studio, but it can also be a corner of a friend's apartment, an activity room in an elderly-care facility, or a row of easels in a preschool. A studio is any place or space where we make art. It is often thought of as a special room, but it can be many different environments—a wall, a kitchen table, or even a laptop sketchbook and a basketful of stimulating materials. It can be portable and can even be a state of mind that you tap into whenever you want to engage the creative source within.

A studio is really a form of sanctuary, making a place for your soul's creative work. Sanctuary is considered a consecrated place or the most sacred part of a religious building. It is also a space that provides protection, spiritual rejuvenation, and solace.

A sanctuary for making art has two basic intentions. The first is practical: space to work, store, and organize creative activities. The second is ambience. The emotional feeling of your studio space reinforces and sustains the work you intend to do there. My own studio space is a place I can go to when I need inspiration, guidance, or regeneration. It is this spirit that makes the space a sanctuary. Even if I am too tired to work, it enlivens me through the visual environment I have created.

Finding a Studio in Your Space

Believe it or not, there is always a studio waiting to be found somewhere in your environment. For an entire year while I was a student at the School of the Museum of Fine Arts, I had a very tiny one-room flat in Boston's North End. My twin bed literally took up most of the room. The only real space I had was a short hallway that led into the space, so I made the back of my front door my studio. It provided a large surface to tack up paper or canvas, and it was conveniently close to my art-supply storage in the bathroom. A small porch on the other end of the flat became home to sculptures or messy projects. I made several hundred drawings and paintings in that space (which were eventually stored under the bed), never really wanting for a bigger space. I learned by necessity that even the smallest environment can be transformed into a studio with care and intention.

During the many years I have worked with groups, my resourcefulness in changing non-art spaces into studio spaces has been repeatedly tested. At times, it seems as formidable as spinning straw into gold, but no matter what the space, I am confident it can be transformed into a place to make art. When I taught at an alternative high school many years ago, my first assignment was to develop an art space for a group of twenty adolescents. Most of the rooms in the school had to be used for several different functions each day. My art room was also used by the Spanish class and counselors who met with students, and in the early morning served as a community space where students and teachers could have coffee and doughnuts. Despite the constant flow of activities through the space, when art class started, the room was automatically transformed through materials, art making, and creativity energy.

Since that time I have facilitated art groups in kitchens, TV lounges, hotel conference rooms, basketball courts, and recreation rooms (where the Ping-Pong table doubles as an art table). At other times, I have had to make do with an office used by a psychologist, where a desk becomes an art space, or transform a patient's hospital room by making a bed tray a space for image making. Part of the pleasure of having a sanctuary is the inventiveness that goes into finding and creating it. Yours may be an old door or board leaned against a wall or a hall table under a skylight. Claim a room in your home or stretch your imagination and carve out a spot that will become your sanctuary for expressive work.

Creating and Nurturing Your Sanctuary

Transform your space into a sacred space. Thinking and intending that a space in your home or workplace is a sacred space sends a powerful message to yourself that creativity is welcome and you are called to express yourself. In one group I facilitate, we light a set of votive candles and bless the meeting room by burning sage at the beginning of each session. A collection of sacred objects that group members selected surround the candles: an animal bone; an image of Kali, the Hindu goddess of life and death; a small Navaho ceramic pot; prayer beads from Japan; and photographs of people with personal significance to individuals in the group. Lighting the candles and seeing the objects is a way for the group to set the mood for artistic expression and reinforce their intentions for creativity.

Make your space special with objects that you love and that hold meaning for you and support your intentions for creative expression. A studio sanctuary is a place in which you feel safe, happy, and nurtured and where you receive the inspiration not only to make images and objects but also to care for the soul. Consider adding any of the following to your studio space:

- Music or chimes for sound
- Natural objects such as stones, feathers, tree branches, flowers, or plants for a connection to nature
- Flowers, aromatherapy burners, incense, or candles for scent
- Fabrics for texture and pattern
- Toys, masks, plastic animals, or other playful memorabilia for the spirit of whimsy
- Prisms or mirrors for reflection and refraction of light
- Reproductions of art, postcards, or other images that inspire creativity
- Photographs of family or people you admire for connection to community

Create an altar or assemblage of images and objects. The way you arrange your materials can be an assemblage that inspires and stimulates your creativity. You may want to collect and arrange objects that hold significance to you or those that simply give you pleasure. I like to create altars in any space where I plan to do creative work. A friend of mine has a small sculpture created by a close friend who died as a reminder of artistic intention and the enduring creative spirit. Others, like the group described above, assemble a collection of objects from nature or home as a reminder of their intentions for art making as a wellness practice. Think of possible compositions you can create with objects that hold meaning for you, and take some time to make a special arrangement of these objects within your studio space.

Treat your supplies with care and mindfulness. Part of the joy of connecting to the soul's palette is keeping your tools and materials in good condition. Caring for the things you use to make art is an act of caring for yourself as well as tending to your sanctuary. Arrange your paintbrushes, pencils, and pens in simple glass jars like bouquets of flowers. Give yourself permission to buy some attractive baskets and boxes to store collage materials, glue, tape, and paint tubes. Clean your brushes, store your papers, and put the lids back on the glue and paints. Tending to your supplies with mindfulness prepares you for creative work and nourishes the source and soul of imagination.

Treat your art with respect. Artists store their work to protect it from damage from light, moisture, or other elements. The most common form of storage is a portfolio, a large, flat folder that generally holds two-dimensional work such as drawings, collages, and paintings on paper; for three-dimensional work such as clay sculpture, a cabinet or shelves may be necessary to keep objects from damage. Treat your work with respect by considering how to store completed works if they are not being displayed. The act of caring for your work is as important as the process of creating it.

Think of your portfolio, box, container, or other storage as an archive of your artistic wisdom. Take out the pieces that you have created from time to time and look at them with a fresh eye. Some may inspire you to develop another drawing or collage, while others may be ready for a new life through the collage box.

Portable Studios

A sanctuary for artistic creativity can consist of items that we take with us as a kind of portable studio. When I was going through a medical crisis, I spent a good part of each week in a doctor's waiting room. I sat in close quarters with ten or fifteen other people in an atmosphere of anxiousness with colorless walls and nondescript furniture. To make the wait more bearable I brought a six-inch-square sketchbook and a handful of colored pencils that fit nicely into a zippered plastic bag in my handbag. Even in the chaos and unappealing surroundings of that waiting room, my six-inch-square territory was a portable studio capable of shutting out everything else. The receptionist usually had to call me several times to get my attention when the doctor was ready for me.

When you attend to your imagination and creative source, you create a special place inside yourself for image work to blossom. The small sketchbook sustained my creativity on most days: at other times when I felt extremely debilitated, my studio was all in my head. I would close my eyes and watch my imagination at work and allow mental images to spontaneously come forth for my entertainment. At other times, simply being outdoors and mindfully looking at leaves, trees, or buildings was my "studio."

Children naturally make portable studios wherever they are. You may have seen a child using a stick to draw in the sand or sinking deep in thought and coloring a picture while sitting with a parent. Children have taught me a lot about how any space can become a studio, no matter how small or unaesthetic. On a cross-country flight recently, I brought a small sketchbook and colored pencils to draw the landscapes or clouds that I might see along the way. I was seated next to two little sisters who were on the way to see their grandparents on the East Coast. Because they were traveling alone, they were understandably anxious about the long flight. While I sat there with my pencils and sketchbook, I could feel the intensity of two pairs of eyes on my coloring.

I offered them some paper and pencils, and they eagerly jumped at the opportunity for something to do. "But what should we draw?" they asked. I suggested, "Well, your grandparents would probably like to know all about your long plane ride today. Maybe you can make them some pictures that tell about your trip." That idea was an immediate hit, and they set about making a series of drawings of the flight attendant, what the pilot might be doing in the cockpit, the horrible meal we had to eat, and what their grandparents would look like when they arrived. We borrowed a stapler from the businessman across the aisle to fasten the pages together. By the end of the trip they had a small book called "The Airplane Trip." They ran to their waiting grandparents at the gate, enthusiastically waving the book they created on the crowded confines of an airplane tray table.

Creative Activities: Making Portable Studio Sanctuaries

Create a movable creative laboratory. My small sketchbook, both in the doctor's waiting room and on the airplane, was a movable creative laboratory for art making whenever or wherever I desired. Your creative laboratory can be a simple sketchpad or journal, a studio that is, aside from some drawing or collage materials, a matter of inches.

Make an Art Rx Box. When I began to bring art to the bedside of a child or adult confined to the hospital, I had to think of a way to transport both materials and a studio to what is usually a very small space. I purchased a plastic file box with a compartment for drawing media, glue, scissors, paper, and collage materials at an office supply store and christened it the "Art Rx Box."

You can make your own Art Rx Box; it can be a box, plastic container, or basket that is portable enough to take with you to your workplace, a hospital waiting room, or the outdoors. Fill it with materials that stimulate your artistic expression and imagination. An Art Rx Box can be an act of service and intention for wellness in others. Think of someone, perhaps a homebound or elderly person or a hospital patient, who would enjoy a portable studio, and make this creative activity a gift to another individual or even a regular practice of inspiring creativity in others.

Find and nurture the studio in your mind. The mind's reality is just as real as what we see and experience in the world. Try using your imagination to create drawings or paintings, or simply to enjoy the experience of touching and handling your favorite materials or colors. Use all your senses when you tap the studio in your mind by imagining what it feels like to use a brush and ink, what oil pastels or tempera paints smell like, or the sounds of clay being slapped on a table. Look around at your environment and see all the possible images that could become future drawings, collages, or clay sculptures. Your imagination is not only a powerful source of creative wisdom, it will also keep you inspired to continue making images.

STARTING OUT ON THE JOURNEY

Now that you know about materials and how to create a studio as sanctuary for your creative source, the following thoughts may be helpful.

Just step on the path. Taking the first step is, at the very least, an intention to expand your vision and do something for yourself. In art making or imaginative work, gathering materials and making plans are acts of hope and can be satisfying in and of themselves. Don't wait until you have more time, the season changes, or the universe gives you a special go-ahead sign. Collect your materials, make marks on paper, feel the texture of clay, and get started.

Make time. You don't have to set aside hours to make art or experience imagination. If you are just beginning, try to schedule three twenty-minute periods a week for artistic expression. You may want to try working first thing in the morning at the breakfast table or as a treat right after dinner. If you set aside a small amount of time for art making, you may find that those twenty-minute sessions are not enough, and you can gradually expand your art-making sessions.

Don't be attached to the outcome. One of the great wonders of art making is that not everything turns out exactly the way we planned. I cannot tell you the number of times in my life that I have not been able to control the paint or I just could not get the colors I wanted onto the paper. These moments seem frustrating, but I relearn how to let go, step aside, trust, and go with the flow. The great thing about art making is that it is the one activity in the world where we can try new things and then discard what we don't want, as many times as is necessary. Out of all the seeds one plants in a garden, only a few may become flowers; what is important is to keep planting.

Clear the space. I find that when I am overwhelmed or confused about the direction I want to take in my creative work or which material to use, or if I feel as if the next image just won't come, I spend some time clearing the space. I wash down my work table; I sort my paper, paints, and brushes; I throw out the dirty water in the glass jars and take an inventory of the collage box. This is a form of practice in itself, a cleansing of both mind and work space. Some image or idea may come to me in clearing out the distractions, or the process of making the space clean and simple quiets my mind. And even if the muses do not visit that day, I am satisfied with the visual pleasure of a well-organized and peaceful environment for the next creative adventure.

Use what you have. While a trip to the art store can be a great adventure that stimulates your creative juices, chances are you have the tools and materials of the soul's palette in your home right now. Look in the junk drawer, use ballpoint pens and #2 pencils, search for images in newspapers and magazines, or consider the materials of nature in your own backyard or neighborhood park as a source of creative expression. Paint with food coloring, draw with lipstick samples you have been hoarding, or sit down with your child and make Play-Doh sculptures. Don't keep waiting for the right materials to appear; start now by using what you have.

Stay on the path of visual imagination and keep making things. The path of visual imagination and art making extends beyond drawing, painting, collage, and clay. You may find yourself drawn to photography, video, or a computer paint program. You may like the tactile qualities of fabric or an art form such as embroidery or weaving. The soul's palette can include what we call crafts, using our hands to create a quilt, decorate a chair, or embellish a favorite shirt. Many traditional and tribal peoples do not differentiate between the idea of art and function. In fact, some cultures do not have a word for art because everything around them is "art," from a handcrafted chair or a carved bowl to an embroidered jacket for a newborn child.

Find those creative activities that match your personality and inspire your artistic expression, but take a risk from time to time and try another medium. When you are able to predict what you are going to do each time you use your artistic creativity, it may mean that it is time for a change. Something as simple as changing materials takes you on an adventure of surprise and mystery, stirs your intuition, and taps the soul's palette in new and exciting ways.

§

The path of art making and imagination is different for each of us. What is important is that you are making images you enjoy making, tapping into your imaginative and visual potential, and infusing creative passion into your life. While specific activities and practices are suggested throughout this book, art making will not transform your life unless you are creating what *you* want to create from the soul's authentic voice. The first steps are finding the materials, creating a sanctuary for creative work, and nurturing ways of making art that please your soul; the rest will naturally follow and flow forth as you continue the journey.

Visual Symbols as Messengers, Guides, and Friends

*T*he symbolic process of artistic creativity is an infinite well from which you can draw insight, self-knowledge, and transformative experiences. Symbols may appear in your dreams or be created consciously. Taking an image from your dreams or imagination and putting it on paper, canvas, or clay enhances your self-understanding and makes visible your personal myths and stories. Symbols in your art may reflect your neglected areas, bring attention to something you need to repair within yourself, or generate the energy needed for change. They naturally tell stories about who you are, where you come from, and where you are going. You never exhaust completely their meanings or healing aspects.

Symbols always carry an element of the mysterious and inexplicable, yet the fact that you can create a symbol through images confirms that fact that you already know the symbol on some level. I believe that the spontaneous, unplanned symbols you dream and create in art help you to find balance and wholeness in your life. They are direct messages from the soul's palette.

Peter London, author of *No More Secondhand Art*, notes that art can be used as the externalized map of our interior self. Artistic expression is an inner source of knowing and I believe that this knowing emerges most clearly when it teaches us in the form of spontaneously created symbols, whether through imagination, dreams, or art making. In this chapter you will learn how to tap your interior self to create spontaneous imagery and to draw from the infinite well of symbols to guide, inspire, and inform your life.

GOING TO THE INFINITE WELL

"Advance confidently in the direction of your dreams," said Henry David Thoreau.[1] It is almost as if the world comes to meet us when we truly follow our inner voices. Sources of help and support, new opportunities, and ideas seem to fall into place when we trust in the process, act with a courageous heart, and travel in the direction of our dreams.

Thoreau's advice suggests that our deepest intuitions are like guides in our lives who are always present; we just need to recognize and cherish them when they come to greet us. Images are one such potent source of guides, whether they are in the form of dreams or images that we collect, meet in the world, or self-create. Dreams, visions, imaginings, and art expression are all conduits for visual symbols. They are messengers of wisdom, beacons in the darkness, teachers, and friends.

The word *symbol* comes from the Greek *symbolon*, meaning token of identity. In ancient times, two friends might break a coin or other significant object when parting; upon returning, the pieces of the object were joined, commemorating the reunification of the parted friends. The rejoining of the parts is a symbol with deep meaning not only for unity but for transformation.

When we take a symbolic image from our dreams or fantasies and transform it into a drawing or object, we put it into concrete form. Once it is realized on paper, canvas, or clay, the image can be witnessed and used to increase understanding of ourselves and our personal myths and stories. This symbolic process is a way for us to experience insight and wholeness and strive for balance and well-being in our lives.

CALLING FORTH SYMBOLS IN ART, DREAMS, AND LIFE

James Hillman says our images are our keepers, as we are theirs. While we are the containers for images and imagination, in order to fully experience their wisdom we must actively prepare a space for these visual symbols to emerge through artistic expression, the dream world, and life. In my own life there are vast, dry deserts of time when few images come forward; at other times, everything seems to be falling into place and images flow freely in my art making, dreams, and daily experiences. Certain states of knowing seem to invite these images to come forth: a sense of intuition, the practice of intention, and attention to synchronicity.

Intuition

Intuition is a natural ability; a means of discovery, problem solving, and decision making; and a key part of the creative process. Not so long ago it was believed to be experienced by only a gifted few. Now it is recognized as something available to everyone and a skill anyone can cultivate. It is not rare or accidental but is something we can call on in everyday life.

Intuition is a form of what physicists call nonlocal reality—a reality beyond the physical (local) realm of the senses, where ideas, thoughts, feelings, and sensations are known instantly. An answer to a problem may appear out of the blue, and an unexpected event or experience may lead us to a new awareness. When we enter nonlocal reality, rules of expression and understanding change. In many traditional cultures of the world, such nonrational ways of knowing the world are accepted as truth. In some cultures, dreams represent literal rather than symbolic reality and are treated as real and tangible. For example, American Indians receive guidance from ancestors, spirit guides, and totem animals. Intuitive images are respected for the knowledge they contain.

Art is an intuitive activity; when working from an authentic and spontaneous place, we make choices about colors, forms, and materials that we are attracted to. This process is a source for cultivating intuition, and the more you notice and practice it, the more present it becomes. When we are able to call on intuition and combine it with creative work, we have the opportunity to bring forth images and symbols that deliver guidance from the soul's palette. Despite the constant availability of intuition, we sometimes find it difficult to access because it comes from a place of mystery beyond the conscious mind. Sometimes it whispers its wisdom, and at other times it bellows at us to trust in what we believe and in what we feel we must do. When intuition calls you, you are being asked to use your creativity and imagination to understand and embrace its message.

There are many ways that you can cultivate your intuition in art making:

◆ Suggest to yourself that you will be aware of those times that you know something intuitively. In painting, drawing, or other creative activities, try to be aware of those moments when the process naturally flows and your hands know just what line to make or color to use.

◆ Pay attention to those times when your hunches are correct and note whether or not you decide to follow your intuition. We learn as much about our intuition when we don't follow it as when we do. Think about what your intuition tells you and when you risk using it and when you do not. Increasing confidence in your intuitive side can become a powerful resource in tapping your inner creative wisdom, consciously or unconsciously.

◆ Art making is a way of cracking the code of intuitive knowing. Think of pencils, crayons, clay, and collage as the technology of intuitive knowing and your imagination as the fuel that feeds this technology. Try practicing this idea by reading it or saying it out loud once a day for a month and especially before creative expression.

◆ Try the following affirmations to help reinforce the importance and power of intuition as a source of knowing:
  • My intuition is my life, dreams, and image making.
  • My intuition supports my well-being and nourishes my soul.

- My intuition helps me in creative, positive, and constructive ways.
- I invite intuition into my life to help me achieve my goals.

Intention

Gary Zukav, author of *The Seat of the Soul*, explains that intention is not only your desire to do something; it is the use of your will. An intention is simply a plan, aim, purpose, or meaning. It can be as simple as having the courage to experiment with materials, or it may be a desire to deepen, through art making, your understanding of a problem you are confronting.

Intention along with art making is a powerful combination. An intention is a conscious action to set a goal or a purpose for your creative work. Formulating an intention helps the mind to focus and can reduce blocks or resistance you may have when undertaking creative work. Because your intentions form the reality you experience, the intention to tap and develop your soul's palette will naturally help you enhance your creative resolve.

A friend told me the following story that weaves together the practice of intention with the power of visual imagination. Her lease on her apartment was expiring, and she knew she had to move in the next month. She lived in an urban area where it was very difficult to find an affordable rent. She really wanted a place with two bedrooms, one of which she could use as a studio, and an eat-in kitchen and a living room with a fireplace. For three weeks every night she went to bed and envisioned her dream apartment, putting out her intention to the universe. She imagined herself walking through the rooms of her new place, seeing her studio, living spaces, and eat-in kitchen. One day on her way home from work, she saw an older woman putting out a "for rent" sign on the front lawn of a two-story home. It turned out that the woman was looking for a tenant for the first floor of her home— with two bedrooms, an eat-in kitchen, and a living room with a fireplace. The rent was within the price range my friend could afford, and the next week, just before her lease ended, she moved in.

Later, she told me something amusing about her new place that happened in the process of visualizing and creating an intention for her dream apartment. It seems that in all those intentions for her new flat, the one thing she neglected to intend was a fire in the fireplace. As it turned out, the new apartment's fireplace was closed off and inoperable. We chuckled, acknowledging that sometimes you do get exactly what you intend, no more and no less!

Setting an intention can help you to get the most from art making and imagination. An intention is a transformational practice because you must make it a part of your life in order for its power to emerge. Try any of the following affirmations on a daily basis:

- I intend to use my creative source to find joy and satisfaction through art making.
- My intention is to express the truth of how I feel.
- I intend for my body to communicate through my drawings.
- My intention is to embrace and celebrate the artist within me.
- I intend to receive the wisdom of my soul's palette.

You may have even more specific intentions for art making and may formulate statements for your creative work such as, "I want to understand why my daughter and I are fighting." Or, "I intend to understand why I am not happy with my career." It is also helpful to write out a statement of your intention. Write it on a piece of paper and keep it in a place in your studio space where you can see it. You may also want to say it out loud and repeat it.

I believe that intention is a powerful tool in using the soul's palette for health and well-being. In any form of transformation, the power of change comes from intention.

Think about what you would like to get from art making in your life. This can be as basic as exploring new experiences with drawing or painting, using art making in your life as a way of reducing stress, or enhancing your sense of wellness through creativity. You can make an intention to increase your understanding of how you express yourself through images, or to know more about how your feelings and life experiences are reflected in art. Your intention may change, but whatever it is, it is important to identify your intentions for art making.

Sometimes an image or symbol emerges unexpectedly in many parts of your life. This experience is often referred to as synchronicity, the appearance of symbols that may take on a magical, mysterious, or even mystical importance over time. A friend related a story that explains how synchronicities may often take years to unfold:

> Yesterday I had a dream of a black face and a white face kissing, joined by a pair of red lips. Remarkably, later in the day someone e-mailed me, saying I might like to look at her friend's website of jewelry, calligraphy, and other design work. When I looked at the site, I was astonished to see a drawing of a black face and a white face sharing the same pair of red lips.
>
> About five years ago I witnessed an extraordinary sight outside of my second-story window: a black crow and a white seagull fighting in midair. It seemed like a significant omen, though what the significance was, I couldn't have told you then. As it has turned out, over these five past years I've grown in my ability to tolerate the conflict of opposite feelings within myself. My dream of yesterday, with the red lips, seems to show a new stage of this black/white process. The synchronicity of seeing the image on the website underlined the importance of my dream symbol and affirmed my intuitive interpretation of it.

You may feel that the recurrence of an image is beyond coincidence, that there is a deeper reason for its repeated appearance in your life. Exploration through art can be a way of knowing all there is to know about your synchronistic symbols and why you are encountering their presence not only in art but in your relationships, work, and other aspects of life.

Although no one really understands how synchronicity happens, most accept without question that it does exist. It also seems that the more we pay attention, the more likely we find synchronicity occurring. What distinguishes synchronicity from coincidence is its meaningful

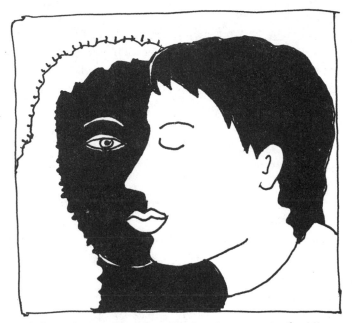

A dream image of two faces sharing the same pair of red lips.

nature. For example, if you suddenly get an unexpected telephone call from someone whom you need to ask a question, then synchronicity is at work.

When we use art with intention, synchronicity is often activated in meaningful ways. Art and imagination help us to let go of linear thinking and open us to nonlocal experiences. They also encourage us to be more fluid and pliant in our thinking, allowing us to enter a realm governed by different possibilities.

When symbols come our way and just won't let go, it is particularly important to pay attention because they may be unrecognized signs of synchronicity in our lives. Sometimes these symbols stubbornly repeat themselves until we recognize and embrace their meaning. Years ago I had an experience that convinced me of the synchronistic potential of personal symbols. After several months of feeling creatively blocked and depressed by a series of life events, I decided to try to break my creative drought by working with papier-mâché sculpture, something I had used as a child in grade-school art classes.

From simple newspaper strips and wallpaper paste, I created a series of seven oval shapes. After they dried, I painted them black, a predictable choice to match my dark mood. They lay on the table in my studio for several days until my husband remarked, "Why do you have all those dead birds in your studio?" I laughed, realizing those black forms did indeed look like black birds lying on their backs. I was also intrigued that perhaps I had found an important image after months of not being able to create. I went on to add feathers and beaks to the forms, making seven dead crows that I laid to rest in a large plexiglass coffin I had had constructed for them at a local glass shop.

My dead crows were only the beginning of a series of black-bird encounters that lasted for the next three years. Several months later, when I was a visiting professor in an unfamiliar town, the taxi driver could not find the address of the place I was to stay. He stopped at three establishments to ask directions: the Club Raven, the Blackbird Restaurant, and a store named Something to Crow About! Either the driver was surely playing a trick on me or this town had an unusually high number of businesses named after black birds. Over the following weeks and months, more crows appeared. At an outdoor market a large crow landed on a car trunk in front of me, pecking at a license plate that read "Be Present." On a trip to an oceanfront boardwalk, a crow flew out of the sky and sat next to me on a bench as if we had known each other for years. Friends who did not know about my crow encounters suddenly sent me greeting cards adorned with ravens and blackbirds.

While I was teaching a group of graduate students at an urban university the following summer, a crow appeared outside the classroom

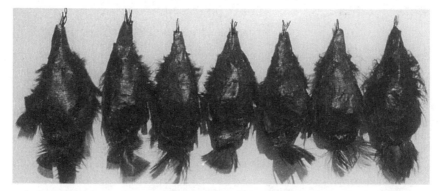

Seven Dead Crows, papier-mâché sculptures by the author.

window, pecking at the glass. I knew by now that it was important to pay attention to this image that appeared with great regularity. I finally excused myself to the class, went to the window, opened it, and asked the crow, "Who are you and what do you want?" My students were amused by their professor who talked to birds, but at that point I knew that these events were important symbols that could not be ignored.

There were more crow encounters in the months to come, and I began to explore the image through art and journaling. I drew and painted a series of crow visitations and came to realize that their stubborn recurrence was a much-needed guide and, later, a companion through a difficult time in my life. At first, the image came to mark an ending phase in my life and a transition to new relationships and work opportunities. But in the end, the experience also led me to learn other lessons: to live mindfully, pay attention, and, in particular, be present to images in my life.

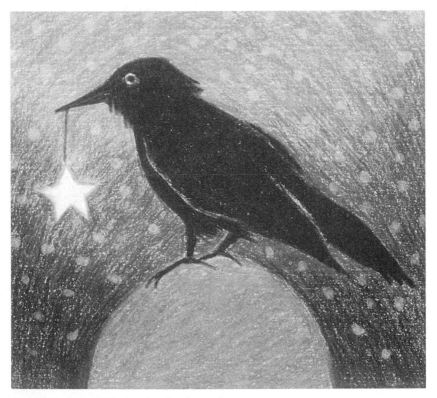

Crow Bringing a Gift, drawing by the author.

Synchronistic messengers, guides, and teachers in the form of symbols come to us most freely and easily when we are unencumbered, open, and authentic. They often seem to be found not through a struggle with materials or process but through surrender to what is joyful and uplifting. Art making allows us to give in to the mystery, through which we renew our connection to feelings of both wonder and well-being. In art making we cannot fully control what will happen or where it will take us. This surrender of will through the creative source is a form of grace in action, an experience that often leads to synchronistic encounters in life and art making.

I have been fortunate to witness this form of grace within myself and many times in the creative process of others. What is often apparent is how the presence of grace makes way for imagination and creativity to transform and heal. One of the most profound experiences in which I beheld the power of grace at work through image was with Jane, a woman in the last stages of cancer. Jane came to my art therapy practice several years ago because of emotional depression and the physical effects of chemotherapy and radiation treatment. She had used art and poetry in the past as a way to make sense of her illness and now wanted to deepen that process as her cancer became more severe and remission became impossible.

Jane did not see herself as an artist but was aware of the power of her dreams and drawings to guide her through what had become a process of letting go as her body became more debilitated by illness. She believed that art was a blessing in her life that opened her to something beyond herself. I felt privileged to witness the way that Jane's creative source sustained her spirit when, in fact, the physical body was dying. In one of her final meetings with me she shared a drawing of a dream she had had on a previous night, recalling: "In my dream I was walking across a bridge from a place of darkness to a place of sunshine and light. I realized that this was a lot like my experience with cancer and dying—that I may be about to cross from this life into the next, a place of spirit and everlasting life. As I walked across that bridge I was surprised to see at my feet a small box, which I reached down to pick up. The outside was dark, perhaps wood or discolored metal. It was worn and looked very old. But when I opened it, the inside was very different—it was filled with gold and light—beautiful things, perhaps a gift of some sort. And when I awakened I felt very peaceful and very pleased to have found and opened the box."

Later in our session I asked Jane if she had ever discovered or come upon something like the box filled with gold and light in her own life. She grinned at me and said with simplicity: "The cancer—I thought you'd know that." Jane's illness had taught her many lessons and inspired her to live life more fully than before her diagnosis. I believe Jane's own inner grace and authenticity were the conduit to a source of healing imagery that presented itself in her dreams and drawings. Her own journey through years of confronting depression, illness, and now death had brought her to a spiritual wisdom realized by very few. Her creative spirit translated this wisdom and provided the stage for transformation through her dream images. Hearing her story and seeing her drawing allowed me to share her experience of wholeness, despite the painful and difficult circumstances of her life.

Some images, like my black birds, are tenacious and seem to emerge spontaneously in life, dreams, or images. Others, like Jane's dream, emerge when we surrender to the mystery and allow something beyond ourselves to come forth. The soul's palette gives us the chance to welcome synchronicity into our lives and experience our natural source of knowing.

Experiment with tuning in to your inner symbols, and make an intention to allow images to emerge in art, dreams, and life. Consider also how synchronicities both in life events and in imagery in your art and dreams coincide with any intentions you have made. Do your images made with intention to solve a problem or receive an answer to a question support what you want to achieve? Consider creating a synchronicity log as part of your explorations of spontaneous symbols. Try to pay attention to both the unexpected events that bring special meaning to your life as well as the smaller moments of "Aha." Take a few minutes every day to write down any coincidences or synchronicities that have occurred. Are you in the right place at the right time, or do you feel you are completely on the wrong track? Are the images you are attracted to or have created reflective of the events in your life?

If you find affirmations helpful, try one or more of the following as a daily practice for the next month:

- I invite synchronicity into my life, dreams, and image making.

- Synchronicity in my life and creativity supports my well-being and nourishes my soul.

- The images reveal synchronicities in my life in creative, positive, and constructive ways.

- I invite meaningful coincidences into my life to help me achieve my goals.

MAKING SPONTANEOUS IMAGES

While we can intuit, intend, or attract symbols, we can also go on a conscious search for symbols in our lives through art making and imagination. But what if you don't know where to start? Fortunately, there are many easy ways to use spontaneous art making to help bring personal symbols to the surface. These are deceptively simple activities that not only are fun but also naturally tap into the creative source. Working spontaneously helps us to be present, mindful, and authentic. Through this type of expressive work you can cultivate your intuition, invite synchronicity, and open to the healing powers of the soul's palette.

Leonardo's Device

Leonardo da Vinci, the Renaissance artist best known for the *Mona Lisa*, invented a deceptively simple technique that can help you to tap images from the soul's palette. The device came to Leonardo one day when he was looking at a wall spotted with stains and cracks. The lines and shapes inspired him to imagine landscapes with mountains, rivers, rocks, and trees, and fantasy scenes with strange figures and faces. Leonardo observed that these random lines and shapes on the wall were like the sounds of bells in whose ringing one might hear any word or name one chose to imagine. What Leonardo discovered was a way to enter and use the unconscious as a creative source for spontaneity, self-expression, and inner knowing.

Leonardo's technique can help you reconnect with your wellspring of intuition and imagination, symbolic and synchronistic images, and your artistic creativity. Even if you have never created with art materials before, three variations of this deceptively simple device will enable you to easily access your ability to create images in powerful and profound ways.

Before starting any of the following activities, take a few minutes to get relaxed and let your mind become quiet. Closing your eyes, listening to relaxing music, or engaging in some form of meditation are good ways to begin using Leonardo's device. If you wish to use intention as part of your art-making process, try including an intention in the form of a statement or question you wish to answer before beginning your creative work.

Variation 1: scribbling like a child. One way to experience Leonardo's device is to return to an activity you probably did as a child—scribbling. As a youngster you scrawled lines on paper with a marker or pen, made squiggles with your fingers in the sandbox at the playground, or created colorful shapes with a large paintbrush at an easel in preschool. Scribbling as you did as a child will help you to create a backdrop for finding spontaneous images much like Leonardo's cracked and spotted walls.

The scribble has been used by psychotherapists as a way to bring unconscious images to the surface. Donald Winnicott, a pediatrician who became known for his psychoanalytic work with children, played a scribble game with his young patients, asking them to create a doodle and then find images within the maze of lines. Others, like pioneering art therapist Margaret Naumburg, was among the first to note that images found in self-created scribbles reflected previously unknown or unspoken thoughts and feelings.

For this activity you will need three sheets of 18-x-24-inch white paper and a set of chalks or oil pastels. Read the entire activity before beginning.

1. Begin by placing a sheet of white paper in front of you on a table or a wall. You may want to tape it to the tabletop or tack it to the wall so it won't move around while you are scribbling.

2. Pick out a single pastel for your scribbles; the color does not matter, but you may want to pick a color other than yellow so that you

can clearly see the lines you make. Place your pastel in the center of the paper, close your eyes, and begin to scribble around the paper. Don't worry if you go off the page; simply make a series of lines for about thirty seconds. If you feel tense, try making a scribble with your hand in the air before you transfer your lines to the paper, or use your nondominant hand to create the scribbles. Repeat this process on each sheet of paper.

3. Stand back and look at the lines and shapes in each drawing to see if you can find an image in at least one of them—a particular shape, a figure, an object—in the scribble. Try turning each drawing around, looking at it from each side. If you made your scribbles on a paper on a tabletop, you may want to hang them on a wall and look at them.

4. Using any colors you wish, fill in an image that you see in one of your scribbles. You can add anything to the image you like or feel is necessary. Think of bringing that image into clearer focus by adding details, colors, and lines.

5. When you are finished, hang your drawing on a wall and allow a title to emerge. Write this on the back of the drawing, along with the date. Complete the remaining two scribble drawings or save them for another session.

Variation 2: scribbling with ink and string. Art therapist Evelyn Virshup developed a scribbling technique comparable to the stained and cracked walls that inspired Leonardo's creativity and artistry. She found that making lines and designs with string dipped in black ink is another way to tap the creative source of spontaneous imagery. I find these scribbles can be particularly stimulating to the eye and inspiring to the imagination. For this activity you will need a bottle of black ink (I recommend water-soluble ink because it is washable), cotton string or yarn, three sheets of 18-x-24-inch white paper, and a set of chalks or oil pastels. I suggest that you work on a flat surface such as a table or the floor in case the ink runs off your paper. Be sure to work on top of newspapers or a table or floor covering because ink can stain surfaces. Also wear old clothing or a smock in case of an accident.

1. Cut a piece of string about 18 inches long. Dip your string into a bottle of black ink; you may have to do this a couple of times to get the string saturated with ink.

2. Drag the string across the paper to make lines, shapes, and textures. By changing your movements, you will create different lines and textures, so try moving the string in several ways: twirl it in a circle, dot it, jab it, wiggle it, or slap it on the paper. The purpose is to fill the paper with lines until you feel that the composition is completed.

3. When you feel satisfied with this ink scribble, go on to make two more ink scribbles on the other sheets of paper. This will allow some time for the first ink drawing to dry.

4. Take the first ink scribble you created and turn it around, upside down, or sideways until you see some image, shape, or form that you like or attracts you. As in the previous scribble exercise, you may see something that looks like a particular object, face, person, animal, or landscape. Using chalk pastels or oil pastels, develop that image, adding whatever you would like to complete the image.

5. Title and date your drawing and hang it on the wall. Complete the remaining two ink scribbles or save them for another session.

Variation 3: paint blots. This activity will help you create images that look similar to the Rorschach inkblot test, which psychologists often use to evaluate personality. While you are not going to be taking an inkblot test, you are going to make your own blots using paint on paper to create spontaneous designs. You will need three sheets of 18-x-24-inch white paper, a set of watercolors (tray or tubes; if you use tubes, place a small amount of each color on a plastic palette or plate), a large watercolor brush, a jar for water, and a set of chalk or oil pastels.

1. Be prepared to work quickly in the first part of this activity. Place the paper and painting materials on a flat, horizontal surface. Be sure to have a large jar of water on hand and readily available.

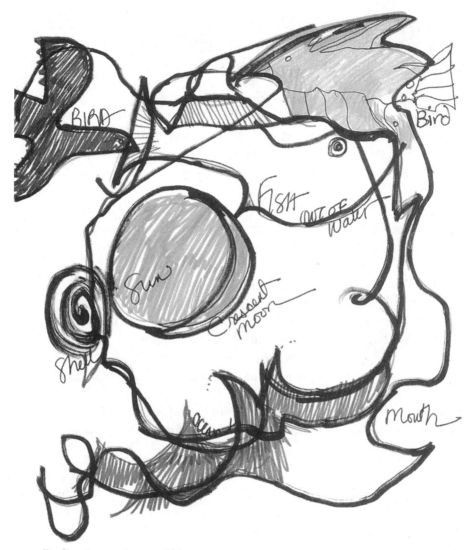

Finding images in a scribble.

2. Dip a large watercolor brush into the water and then dip it into one or more of the colors on your palette or in the tray watercolors. Quickly paint the surface of your paper, filling in most of the paper with color. Before the paint dries, fold the paper in half and rub the back of it with your hand. This will create a paint blot similar to a Rorschach inkblot. Open the paper and allow the paint to dry.

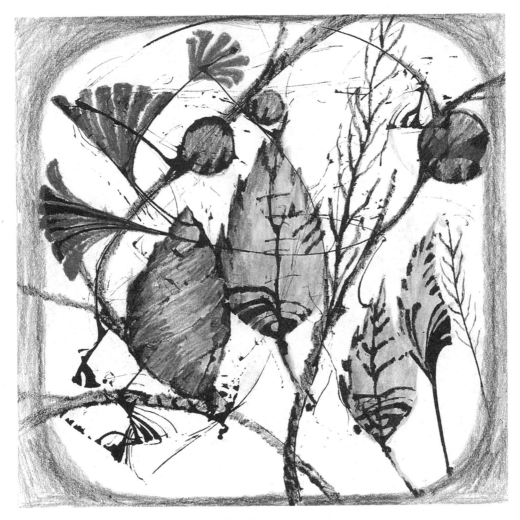

Images discovered in a string scribble by the author.

3. Complete two more spontaneous paintings; by the time you have finished the third painting, your first one should be completely dry.

4. Look at your first painting, turning it sideways and upside down as you did with the previous scribble exercises, until you see some image, shape, or form that you like or that attracts you. As in the chalk scribble exercise, you may see something that looks like a particular object, face, person, animal, or landscape. Using chalk pastels

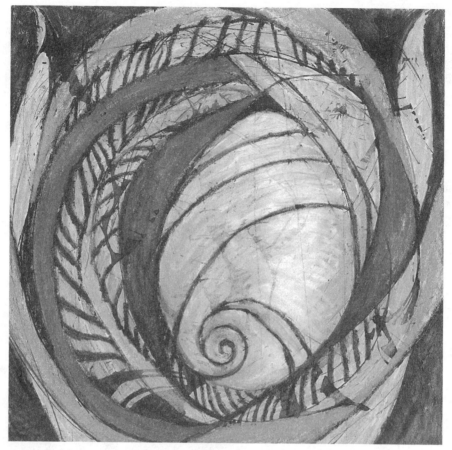

Seedpod, image created from a string scribble by the author.

or oil pastels, develop that image, adding whatever you would like to complete the image.

5. When you feel your drawing is finished, give it a title. Go on and complete the other two paintings or save them for another session.

§

After trying one or more of these variations, you may be surprised by your ability to use your imagination to find images in your marks and lines. Leonardo's device is a way of working with your imagination that is both relaxing and liberating to your artistic creativity. In using these techniques over time as a form of practice, you will become more confident in your creative source and nurture your intuition, and you may evoke synchronicities through symbolic expression.

You may want to write about or talk with the images you have created in any of these activities to understand their messages and wisdom; ways to do this are more fully described in the next chapter. Remember to date each drawing so you will be able to keep track of the order in which you created them. For now it is important that you simply develop your spontaneity and imaginative powers. As you work with these techniques over a few weeks, the content of your drawings will naturally evolve, symbols and patterns will emerge, and your visual vocabulary will increase.

Touch Drawing

On the last day of the last year of artist Deborah Koff-Chapin's study at Cooper Union in New York, she came upon a spontaneous way of drawing that tapped the depths of her soul. She was helping a friend clean an inked glass plate with a paper towel in the print shop when her fingers began to make lines across the back of the towel. She lifted the paper towel from the plate and discovered that her fingers had made a drawing that had been transferred to the underside.

Koff-Chapin was profoundly moved by the directness and spontaneity of her drawings. These "touch drawings" not only were reflections of her soul but also recorded her soul in motion and in continual transformation. She was so deeply struck by the experience that she continued to explore this way of drawing for over two decades, teaching it to others with the aim of finding wisdom and creativity through the process.

Touch drawing is a special form of what is known as monoprinting, a process in which a single unique print is created from a printing plate. The basic materials needed are a tube of printing ink or oil paint (there are water-soluble oils that wash off very easily); a soft rubber brayer to roll out the ink; a piece of plexiglass; and lightweight paper such as tissue paper or newsprint. Do not use acrylic paint for this activity, as it dries too quickly.

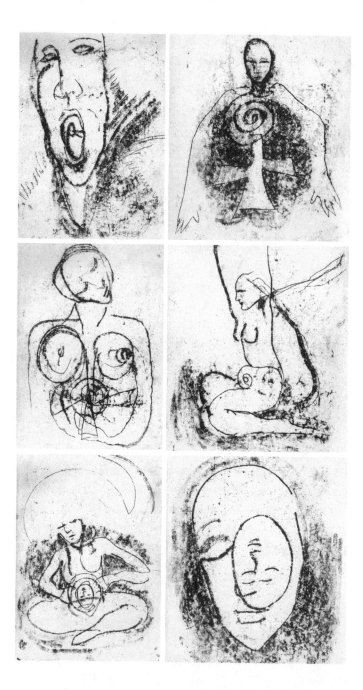

Birth Series © 2001 Deborah Koff-Chapin. "These Touch Drawings are selections from a series done during contractions while giving birth," she says. "Creating with the pain rather than just bearing it transformed my experience of labor."

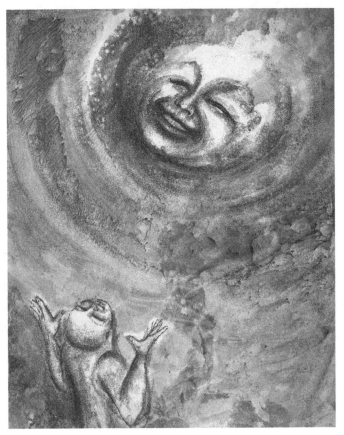

Soul Card © 2001 Deborah Koff-Chapin. "Touch Drawing can be used for the expression of joy as well as pain. This one was done during a meditation retreat."

1. Start by putting some paint on the plexiglass. Use the rubber brayer to roll out the paint until you have a smooth, thin layer on the plexiglass.

2. Place a sheet of paper over the plexiglass; if the paper absorbs too much paint, try blotting off the excess with the paper and place another clean sheet of paper over the painted plexiglass.

3. Koff-Chapin suggests that you turn inward and become aware of any body sensations, feelings, or thoughts before you begin to draw. Take some time to become still and become open to the process. You may also make an intention in the form of a statement or question before beginning.

4. There are a variety of ways to begin drawing. Try closing your eyes and simply moving both hands, including you fingers and fingertips, across the paper. Make gestures, allow your fingers to dance, or find a rhythmic motion for both your hands simultaneously. When your drawing feels complete, remove the paper from the plexiglass and place another piece on the surface; you can usually use the same paint for several drawings.

5. Let your drawings dry, but remember or record the order in which you completed them. It may become important later to recall how images emerged and in what sequence.

Touch drawing can become a transformational practice if you decide to engage in it on a regular basis. Use it along with meditation and music to deepen your experience with creating spontaneous images through your fingers and hands. For Koff-Chapin it has been a lifelong practice that has yielded thousands of drawings and two sets of what she calls Soul Cards (see resources for more information); these cards contain wonderful images that will engage your imagination, intuition, and synchronicity.

Other Ways to Evoke Spontaneous Images

You can also keep your spontaneous imagination flowing with these simple activities:

◆ Place white paper near a window and let the shadows of tree branches, plants, or objects fall onto the page. Freely trace these shadows with a pencil, pastel, or pen; use your nondominant hand if you wish. See what emerges in the lines and shapes.

◆ Scribble on self-stick notes, a notepad, or small scraps of paper while you are talking on the phone. Keeping your conscious mind occupied with conversation will help you to access your spontaneity through your doodles. Use a ballpoint pen and simply make marks and lines all over each paper as freely as possible.

◆ Here's a device that many artists use to find compositions. Cut a 2-inch-square window in a piece of cardboard and look through it at objects around you. Look at a tree trunk and notice the lines in the bark. Hold up your window to look at a section of the clouds, or like Leonardo da Vinci, study a section of an old wall for shapes and cracks. Use your imagination to find images, and write descriptions and titles for them.

TAKE IMAGES AS THEY COME

Sometimes an image that is present or recurring in our lives is the best place to start. Try the following activity as a form of spontaneous image work:

1. Look around for an object or image that evokes a feeling in you. It can be a plastic animal or figure, a postcard image, a picture from a calendar, or a found object. If you don't have an object or image immediately on hand, try letting one come to you. Take a walk down a city street, go to the park, or clean out a closet and see what you find; you might open today's mail and receive a card from a friend with a compelling image on it. Sometimes it is best to just wait for an object or image to present itself to you. This may bring about a synchronicity, and the coincidence of the symbol that presents itself to you can be very important.

2. Once you have found or identified your object or image, meditate on its qualities. Take some time to quiet yourself and simply be with the object or image. Write down a description of this object/image—its colors, textures, forms, and elements—and also any thoughts or feelings that come to mind. Make a drawing of your object/image—draw it as an abstract, draw it as a child would, change its colors to suit your mood, add other elements that seem appropriate, make it big or make it small.

3. If you are more comfortable writing about it, think about the following questions, writing your responses in your journal:

- Why did you choose this symbol? Why did this symbol come into your life?
- How did you come upon this symbol?
- Does this symbol have a personal significance to you?

- What symbols guide your life right now (personal, spiritual, etc.)?
- What symbols have you inherited from someone else (a person, a community, a culture)?
- Are there other symbols currently coming into your life? What are they? Are they related to this symbol in some way?

IMAGE JOURNALS:
A TRANSFORMATIONAL PRACTICE

Jung made a practice of drawing spontaneous images in a journal every day. He believed that these images arose from his inner world and that they were sacred symbols of his higher self. You can engage in the same transformational practice and record spontaneous images, develop intuitive knowing, and explore synchronicity.

Your image journal can take many forms. It can be as simple as a notepad or sketchbook, a bound book, or a self-created journal in a style and format that suit your creative expression. You may want to use it on a daily basis as a visual diary of impressions, feelings, dreams, or events, or you can use it just when you feel the need to. Or you may want to use it in a more specific way or with a specific intention for understanding, resolution, or wellness. Jung's drawing journal is a wonderful example of art making with intention. In Jung's case, his intention was to express through image his journey to his higher self.

An image journal is a good place to begin using your soul's palette for wisdom and wellness but it is also is an intention to commit to image making. Over the last two decades I have been keeping image journals with various themes and formats, to understand and explore my feelings; to work toward a goal, artistic or otherwise; to solve problems with relationships and work; and to enhance my sense of well-being when physically ill. I have also used them as a place to express myself in a spontaneous, uncensored way and, in doing so, have supported my intuitive wisdom and increased my understanding and recognition of synchronistic symbols in my art and dreams.

Be sensitive to your own needs in choosing or designing your journal. The type and size of notebook you use should fit your preferences for format and materials. Sometimes you may want something that fits into your handbag or briefcase, so you can carry it with you and work with it any time during the day. Do you like a large page where you can cut loose, or do you find yourself wanting the security of a small, square paper? If you work in your journal mainly at home or in your studio space, you might want a larger format. If you want something more portable, then a smaller journal may be the best choice.

Timing is also important. For me, image journaling seems to come in cycles. Several of my journals over the years are half full because I grew tired of the paper or the size of the book. Sometimes I just wanted to start over. Other times I wanted a notebook that allowed me to remove or replace sheets. I think literally and symbolically I wanted to say, "This chapter of my life is finished, I am starting over again." I kept several image journals after a personally significant trip to Asia but found by the middle of the third one I just didn't have anything more I needed to express about my experiences. You may find that suddenly a particular journal you have started no longer appeals, while another one beckons you.

An image journal can begin with a ballpoint pen, some magazine photos, and an unlined notepad. Later, you can glue these images into a bound or spiral sketchbook. An artist friend keeps her image journals in binders and buys different colored papers at a stationery store. Make your journal special by decorating the covers with pictures, postcards, fabric, dried flowers, or self-created images. What is important is that you choose what is right for you and have fun.

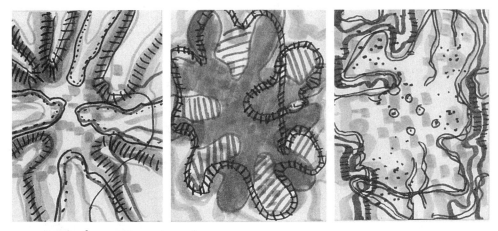

Entries from an image journal.

The following supplies are helpful in starting an image journal:

- An artist's hard-bound journal, drawing pad, or spiral sketch-book of any size; but 11 x 14 inches is a good dimension for most work
- Colored pencils, water-soluble crayons, colored marking pens, and/or oil pastels in 24-color sets
- Watercolors and brushes
- Acrylic or tempera paints and brushes
- Collage materials such as photo images, colored papers, and magazines
- White glue and scissors for collage work

In beginning an image journal, think about your work one page at a time. If using a bound book seems like an overwhelming commitment to filling all the pages with images, begin with a single page. You can keep your images in a folder or portfolio. Make a series of minicollages on unlined filing cards. Take the self-stick notepad drawing activity described in chapter 4 (page 57) and extend it into the transformational practice of image journaling. Keep a Post-it note doodle journal at home or work; use it to make spontaneous, uncensored images whenever you have time or feel the urge. You can even start by coloring the squares of your calendar each day, if that feels comfortable. Any series of images can be your image journal. Don't let size or quantity be intimidating factors.

§

Now that you know how to access symbols as messengers, guides, and teachers, it is time to deepen your experience through discovering their meanings. In the next chapter, you will find a variety of ways that you can enter images, learn their stories, and tap their wisdom for health and well-being.

SIX

Letting Your Images Tell Their Stories

The soul's palette is a form of internal guidance designed to illuminate your way through life. However, to access that inner wisdom, we not only have to make an opening for our images to come forth; we also have to actively translate this wisdom through exploring their stories and meanings. Your artistic creativity helps you to express feelings, memories, and experiences and naturally helps you to visualize the meaning of what is within. But in order to fully tap the healing potential of the soul's palette, we often have to ask our images to speak their truths by giving them a voice.

This chapter explains ways you can talk with your images, how to develop narratives through creative dialogue or writing, and how to use techniques such as active imagination to add meaning to your creative process. You will learn to experience your personal symbols "multimodally"—in other words, through using music, movement, and writing to illuminate the knowledge of the soul's palette. You will also learn how you can use personal and universal wisdom to find meaning for your symbols to enhance your understanding of images in art and dreams. By the end of this chapter, you will have a variety of techniques at your disposal to help you create meaning for your artistic expressions and enhance your experience with your creative source.

ART AS STORY, METAPHOR, AND SYMBOL

Visual images have always been an important part of communication and were used as words in many cultures, preceding writing. Hieroglyphics of the ancient Egyptians, cuneiform scripts of the Sumerians, and contemporary Asian characters are examples of images as language. The use of image as word began art's long history as a way to tell stories.

By nature, we are storytelling beings. To be a human is to have a story to tell. The images we create are the reflections of ourselves and our experiences, and contain the stories of our lives. As an art therapist I see part of my work as helping people use art to express and, in some cases, rewrite their stories, whether those stories are about illness, losses, transitions, or awakenings. Without stories, we cannot make sense of things. As an artist, I see art making as a way to tell me where I am in my own life story. It also helps me to revise the plot as new experiences come along or when I learn new lessons about myself. We all can make meaning through images to tell stories that are inexpressible through words alone. And, in turn, images can help us to make changes in our lives if we spend some time exploring their stories.

Because art does not have rules of grammar, structure, or syntax like spoken and written language, its messages are not always crystal-clear. Images are sensory in their nature and thus serve as metaphors rather than literal representations of ideas, experiences, and feelings. While images may have specific meanings we can easily recognize, their real power is found through the metaphors and symbols within them.

Working with metaphor involves the skill of transforming one thing into another thing that is more valuable. Metaphors are intimately connected to the concept of transformation; in ancient Greek, the word *metaphor* means a transformer. Children naturally transform so many things they encounter around them. With imaginative boldness, they turn bed pillows into mountains, a cardboard box into a ship, and a blanket into an ocean to sail across. Like children, we need to use the power of metaphor to touch the inner truths of the images we create, because metaphor is the authentic reflection of artistic creativity. Like art, it is dynamic, has no strict rules about meaning, and is by nature fluid and flexible.

In addition to metaphors, images contain symbols. Visual symbols have been present in all cultures throughout history, from their first appearance in Paleolithic cave paintings to modern civilization. They have been used extensively in art, literature, myths, and rituals and contain specific connotations that may impart universal meanings across cultures and over centuries. Jung observed that symbols possess meanings that may be unconscious or unknown to us but stimulate our interest and challenge us to understand them. Symbols that appear to us through dreams and spontaneous art making may represent something that is unknown or repressed, or that has not reached consciousness.

The symbols we meet in art, dreams, and life can allow us to perceive our experiences in larger, more universal contexts. Making images encourages us to find meaning in our symbols because we can see them in a tangible form and experience their sensory aspects. While our dreams and imagination may contain symbols, our artistic creativity allows us to become a witness to them in a tangible way.

Symbols have a life of their own and an actual life span. There is a time of birth (the origin, creation, or appearance of the symbol); a time of growth (the amplification, exploration, or transformation of the symbol); and the ending (we lose interest in the symbol or another symbol emerges). My encounter with black birds is a good example of this life cycle. The first sculptures of dead black birds I created marked the birth and emergence of this symbol. Initially, they represented the loss and ending of a part of my life; eventually they marked an important transition that I needed to acknowledge and grieve. During subsequent weeks and months the image revealed many other meanings and helped me to learn deeper lessons through its recurrence. Finally, when its meanings and teachings were exhausted, the birds lost their importance, gradually disappearing. The experience taught me something else: as long as a symbol has something to teach us, it stays present in our lives. This is why it is important to spend time with a symbol and to encourage it to develop and flourish.

We can bring symbols to life through images, and we can further understand their messages by writing about them and by using creative modes of expression to help amplify personal meaning. During the time that we work with a symbol it may transform and surprise us with its varied meanings. Often these meanings change over time, and how we see the symbol today is not the same as it will be next week, next month, or next year. In some cases, the symbol may predict where we are going before we realize that we are even on the journey.

When you make an image or encounter one in a dream, you may be tempted to try to interpret it for meaning. First and foremost, it is important to try not to psychoanalyze your art for meaning and implications. Trying to find out what a symbol stands for bypasses the deeper capacity of images to embody inner wisdom and enhance your well-being. Asking an image, "What do you represent?" is not necessarily the best approach to take when working with the imaginal world. Images are like living things. They come from a place of imagination, and in this realm there are special ways to communicate with images that resonate with the creative process and reflect the truth of artistic expression.

USING YOUR IMAGINATION TO FIND MEANING

Your imagination is a powerful way of understanding and making meaning out of your images. It is not only the source from which you create images but also your resource in seeking wisdom from your images. It may tell you where to go next in your creative process, direct you on how to develop your images, or guide you to move on to something new.

The American philosopher John Dewey described imagination as the ability to see the world as if it were otherwise. When we can see things "as if," we encounter them in a different way. When we use imagination, there are no fixed outcomes, but there are infinite possibilities, nonlogical discoveries, and many mysteries yet to be solved. Imagination expresses our sense of adventure, potential, and hope and is guided by a sense of play. When we imagine or see things "as if," we play with connections between images and thoughts. We may see them in contrast, in harmony, or in new and surprising dimensions.

Invented Dialogues

I sometimes have imaginary conversations, in my head or out loud, in which I take both sides of the discussion, talking back and forth with myself. These invented dialogues help me to see other perspectives about people or events in my life. While people around me who hear these conversations may think I am acting strangely, these dialogues involve using my imagination as a way to make new connections.

Having a dialogue with my images is a form of free association for me. Free association has its roots in psychoanalysis as a form of spontaneous expression that generates new connections as well as taps unconscious meaning. In traditional psychoanalysis, the therapist might invite the person to free-associate feelings, fantasies, or perceptions that help to uncover hidden meanings. We can also free-associate with artistic expressions or dreams to recognize their wisdom and reveal content that may not be obvious just by viewing the image.

There are many ways to invent dialogue that helps us to tap the wisdom of our artistic expressions and encounters with images. Try any or all of the following:

Become the image. Try talking from the image as if you were the image, rather than talking about it. Use phrases such as "I am" or "I feel." In other words, instead of saying that your painting has a lot of blue circles in it, you might say, "I am many blue circles and I feel crowded, happy, passionate, and playful." Personify the elements in your images and use them to describe your experiences and perceptions.

Conduct an interview. Treat images as you would people rather than as expressions to analyze and decipher. Talking with an image as you would a person rather than an object reflects more accurately its true meaning and reflects the soul of its creator. Interview your images and ask them questions. If the image could talk to you, what would it say? Pretend that you can animate the image you have created. Look at various parts of your image and give each a voice. For example, if there is blue square in the image, what would that blue square say? Or, if you selected an image of a tree from a magazine for a collage, what would that tree say? Try answering these questions in the first person ("I am a caged tiger and I feel restless"), spontaneously writing down whatever comes to mind.

How do you feel today? I have a tradition of starting children's therapy groups with a question: How do you feel today? While I am interested in hearing in words how each child feels, I also encourage them to show me in a sensory way with colors, shapes, and lines. Look at your images and ask them to tell you how *they* feel right now. You can ask this of a line, a color, an abstract shape, or a figure within the image. When you look at the drawing, painting, or other art expression, a feeling is always conveyed. Rather than intellectually determining or assigning a meaning, try to look at the image for its emotional quality. What are your initial impressions? Is the image happy, angry, sad, or anxious? Or does it have many different feelings expressed through color, line, and form? How did you use color, line, and form to express emotion?

Make another image. Talk to your image by making more images. In a sense, you will be using the language native to the artistic process as your guide. Try using the language of art making as a way to understand and become more aware of your artistic expression. Continue this process as long as you wish or with as many images as you feel necessary.

Active Imagination

Jung proposed a method of working with images called active imagination. He realized through his own experiences with mental images that one had to directly enter into them in order to understand them. He referred to active imagination as dreaming the dream onward, a way of freely associating from the original image experienced in a dream to other images, thoughts, and feelings as they arise.

Active imagination was thought by Jung to tap the universal world of myth and heritage—the collective unconscious and archetypes. The collective unconscious is the part of our psyche that is the seat of instinctive thought and behavior, as shaped by centuries of human experience. Jung observed that it contains primordial images that cannot be brought to consciousness but could be examined in symbolic form such as art or dreams. He referred to these primordial images as archetypes and believed that they were common to all individuals across cultures.

The technique of active imagination can also be used with drawings, paintings, and other art images, helping you to generate a story from your art. It may also be used to generate another series of images. The associations that one makes to a drawing or painting through active imagination are spontaneous and uncensored, and reflect life experiences and perceptions, environmental influences, and universal symbols. In exploring your images through active imagination, you may find that you discover personal associations (meanings particular to you), cultural associations (meanings associated with the environment or culture in which you live), and universal associations in your art and the images, thoughts, and feelings that arise from the process.

The goal of active imagination is to help you explore yourself through metaphor and to develop a spontaneous, personal narrative to enhance understanding, insight, and growth. It underscores that fully understanding images takes time, that images have many meanings, and that interpretation is shaped by personal, cultural, and universal dimensions.

Active imagination generally involves the following steps:

1. Quiet your mind in a similar way to meditation.

2. Allow images to enter your field of attention and focus on them without holding on with too much concentration or allowing images to pass by without observation. This balance between the relaxation needed to allow images to emerge and the tension necessary to attend to the images can be difficult to achieve and may require both patience and practice.

3. Record what has been seen in writing or in an art medium such as painting, to give form to the experience.

4. Reflect on the messages you received from the experience.

Art expression in itself is a form of active imagination. The images that arise from the process of spontaneous drawing, painting, or sculpting provide material that you can amplify through sticking with the image. "Stick to the image" is a phrase used by Jungian analyst Rafael Lopez-Pedraza and James Hillman with reference to dream images. They emphasize that we need to pay close attention to the uniqueness of our images in order to let it tell their stories. By staying with the scene, mood, and context of the image, we are more likely to find its true meaning.

The following story may help you to better understand the process of active imagination and sticking with an image. Jenna, a woman in her late twenties with a history of depression and broken relationships, was able to use drawing as a form of active imagination. Jenna did not feel that she was artistic but kept a drawing and writing journal for many years. I asked her if she would like to learn some techniques that she could apply to her journal work, particularly her interest in drawing. I explained the process of active imagination to her as a way to generate mental images, helped her to practice it, and asked her to try it several times on her own before coming to our next meeting. I also suggested that if she wanted to, she could make a drawing in her journal of the images she saw during active imagination.

Jenna's first active imagination images were of a dark tunnel at the end of which a star emerged. She recorded what she remembered of her initial active imagination experiences as follows: "At first I can only see darkness and then I realize that I am looking through a tunnel. Below me there is water, but I can't see it because it is so dark. Ahead there seems to be a distant light, so I decide to try to walk down the tunnel to reach it. The light seems faint, like a small white light. As I get closer, it seems to reflect on the walls of the tunnel. I begin to see that it is a five-pointed star with many different colors in it, and although it shines strongly, I can see all the patterns in it. Suddenly I feel that I can go no farther and give up trying to see anymore."

In subsequent sessions she used the star image as a starting point for art expression, both during our meetings and at home when she continued her active imagination exercises. By sticking to the image, Jenna was able to amplify her own meanings for her images both through writing about them and by using them to develop more drawings. Her artwork and active imagination experiences eventually reflected a slow transformation from depression to more positive feelings about the future and to understanding how she could change her relationship with her mother to one in which she could feel more autonomy. Simultaneously, the image moved from its original dark surroundings and eventually appeared as a multipointed star alone in the sky.

Jenna was in therapy for several months, and fortunately was committed to staying with the process of active imagination, drawing, and writing, despite severe bouts of depression on many days. Active

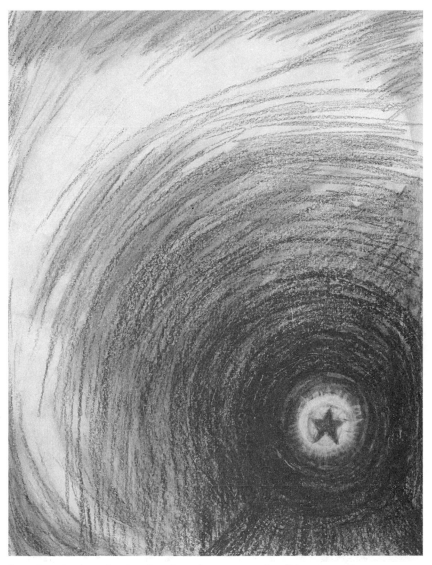

Jenna's active imagination drawing of a star emerging from a tunnel.

imagination requires that you be ready and able to undertake the process of self-examination and expression. In other words, you have to be willing to stay and work with the images that emerge over what may be a long period of time. Jenna was ready to make that type of commitment, and her active imagination work revealed a story of

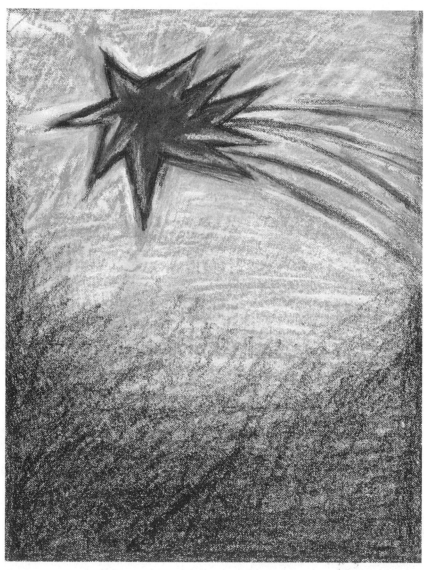

Jenna's multipointed shooting star.

transformation and recovery through both words and images. Sustaining this process is similar to a spiritual practice because it requires regular attention in order to begin to find the meaning and wisdom of your images.

Receptive Imagery

Receptive imagery is another source of imagination and is a technique that involves deep relaxation as a pathway to tapping imagery within. It is imagery that flows through or pops up into your conscious mind; that is, you don't intentionally create it. It often emerges just at the moment you fall asleep or just before you wake up, what are known respectively as hypnagogic or hypnopompic states. Our dreams also seem to be received rather than purposively created.

A simple way to engage receptive imagery is to take some time to relax, focus on your breathing, and turn your attention to the rhythm of your breath. Start to become aware of your body, moving your mind's eye to different parts in turn—the top of your head, the back of your neck, and so on. Be open to any sensations like temperature, tightness, pain, or tingling. Do any colors, shapes, or images come to mind? Anything that comes into your mind during this brief visualization is receptive imagery.

The process can be as simple as imagining yourself in a pleasant environment or it may involve a series of specific elements. Some of the many specific visualizations that are available on tape take you on a journey where you encounter obstacles, meet a guide or teacher, or find an insight, gift, or answer to a question. Others encourage you to develop your own imagery, particularly images that are calming or healing to body, mind, and soul. For example, you might be directed to imagine being bathed in warm, golden light or remember a positive memory with loved ones or friends.

While visualization is a way to generate imagery and use your imaginative capacity, it is also a way to deepen your understanding of your own self-created images. Try working with your art expressions in a receptive way. Take a little while to relax, rest your attention on your breath, and concentrate on the content of your creative work. Be open to any sensations in your body and to any mental images that come to mind. If a visual picture does not come to mind, perhaps you sense something through movement, sound, taste, or smell. Write down these observations, make a sketch in your image journal, or use this receptive imagery as the inspiration for another drawing, painting, or sculpture.

Writing

Writing about your creative work gives images a context and grounds them in time and space. It serves as a record of events, feelings, and experiences associated with the image and is a way to witness your work. Writing about your images on a regular basis, especially during times of stress, is a wellness practice that is both health giving and anxiety reducing.

If you are working in an image journal, at least title each piece and write a few phrases about your images, such as your impressions or feelings, associations, or simple descriptions of colors, lines, shapes, and content. If nothing comes to mind, put your images in a place where you can see them every day. After a short time, a connection or insight will naturally emerge. Record this in writing, either on the back of the picture or in a separate notebook.

While I am not suggesting that you use writing to "analyze" your images, I believe that it can be very important to write something about your visual work, even in the form of short phrases. This simple act may help you to understand, over time, what your images mean personally to you. You will undoubtedly find that when you look back over both your images and your writing that patterns, connections, and new ideas emerge.

Creative writing, in the form of prose or poetry, deepens the experience of image making and stimulates your creative source in a way that art cannot. Try writing a story about a drawing or collage or expressing your thoughts about a painting through haiku. Gabriele Rico, the author of several books on creative writing, suggests using word sculptures as a way of combining the visual with narrative. Try rapidly scribbling with a pen across a large paper to reflect your overall felt sensation in the moment. After you finish, fill it in with colors, words, and phrases. The shapes and colors add to your design and become both a visual and a verbal metaphor of your thoughts and feelings. Continue the process as long as you like or with as many word sculptures as you like.

Intermodal Work

While most ways of tapping the wisdom of your images involve talking or writing, you can use other art forms as ways of exploring and finding meaning. Intermodal approaches rely on a variety of arts as a way to express and deepen understanding of your imagery. For example, rather than using verbal descriptions to explain or describe an image, you respond to it through sound, movement, or acting. Expressive therapists Paolo Knill, Helen Barba, and Margo Fuchs describe dreams as an example of the intermodal qualities of imagination: "Consider dreams, where the soul speaks through imagination. We may sense the movement of swimming or hear a voice or speak words; we may experience the act of killing or see a beautiful visual image of a city, or listen to the sound and rhythm of music."[1]

Working intermodally you might use any of the following approaches:

Music. Don Campbell, author of *The Mozart Effect*, reminds us that music, singing, chanting, and other forms of sound are expressions of our emotions. It is well known that sound and music have powerful effects on our minds and bodies. Music can evoke feelings and memories, and can stimulate the soul's palette.

Experiment with sound, music, and silence as elements in your creative process. Humming a favorite tune, listening to a tape of shamanic drumming, or chanting a series of words may stimulate your creative flow or deeply relax you while you are working. After you complete a painting or drawing, try finding the rhythm of the lines, shapes, and colors within it. All art has the element of rhythm in it; try creating a sound or song that describes the essence of your image.

Movement. Movement is an art form that can help you access the energy of your images. Use movement to enact an emotion or experience, to mirror lines, colors, or shapes, or to tell a story. Look for the

movements of lines in your drawings or paintings that appear frequently; use dance to interpret what you see or feel about these movements in your creative work.

Multimodal. Multimodal work refers to combining all art forms—
music, movement, dramatic enactment, writing—to find meaning
for your artistic expressions. For example, you might create a sound
or music to describe an element and then perhaps use movement to
deepen your experience, and then finally write a poem or short story
about your image and creative process. Using all your creative
sources of self-expression through movement, sound, and image is an
opportunity to use the potentials of all your senses to increase your
understanding of symbols and metaphors in your images.

WISDOM TRADITIONS

Over many millennia humans have developed ways of understanding
the wisdom contained in images, whether in the form of dreams, visions, or art. Much of this wisdom is intuitive; that is, it comes from
nonlogical, even mystical sources of knowing. Other wisdom traditions are based on universal symbols, myths and stories, and rituals
that are common to many cultures throughout the world's history.

Use a good symbols dictionary as a way of illuminating your understanding of your images. David Fontana and Barbara Walker have
written several that provide a thoughtful study of symbols in various
cultures. Angeles Arrien identifies five universal shapes—circle, spiral, cross, triangle, and square—that are found in the art of most cultures and in the images of people of all ages. She believes that all
human beings attribute similar meanings to these five shapes. If you
enjoy creating images with one or more of these forms, the cultural
wisdom that Arrien has collected may be useful in your exploration
of the meaning of your work.

If you enjoy reading myths or studying the Tarot or the meaning
of dreams, those fields can also inform your path of discovery. In con-
sulting any wisdom traditions about symbols, remember to use them

as a guide rather than as dogma. Notice what resonates with you personally when you read about symbols and symbolism. The great Persian poet Rumi sums it up nicely: "Don't be satisfied with stories, how things have gone with others. Unfold your own myth."[2] There are many guides to help you find meaning, but you are the only source for your story. The stories embedded in your images will deepen the transformative powers of your creative source and tap the innate wellness within you. Anytime we engage in the creative process of image making or simply encounter images in our dreams, we connect with a personal mythology that we have developed over time and within the culture and events of life. Our ability to create images that tell stories is clearly a capacity to reflect ourselves and the personal stories of our life journeys.

BE PRESENT

Rather than looking for a set of meanings or answers, sometimes simply being present to your images is a way of knowing. I find that the experience of being present to my images is similar to the practice of *vipassana* (insight) meditation. In this form of Buddhist meditation, one finds a place of awareness from which to observe the internal river of thoughts and sensations that flow through body and mind. Being present to your images without getting attached to them is simply seeing and being with them without judgment. As in meditation, the internal "witness consciousness" is strengthened, and you have the opportunity to practice nonattachment to feelings and experiences.

When you practice *vipassana* meditation, you choose an object on which to focus your mind, and this object becomes the center of meditation. Traditionally, the breath is taken as the object. In the simplest form of the practice, you focus on the in-and-out of the breath. Whenever you realize that your mind has strayed from the breath, you simply note that and return your attention to the breath.

While *vipassana* is a path of making meaning through self-observation, being present to images is a way of knowing through observing what has been created by the self.

1. Choose a suitable place for sitting with your image; a place that is secluded and quiet is best.

2. Sit in a comfortable posture without leaning against anything. You can use a well-padded cushion on the floor or a chair. Whatever posture you adopt, make sure that before you begin the meditation proper, it fulfills these three conditions: comfort, a straight back, and easy, natural breathing.

3. Start by keeping your eyes gently closed for a few minutes, and fix your attention on the breathing process. Become aware of the breath as it passes over the upper lip and through the nose. Breathe naturally, just watching the breath as it is. Don't try to control it or change it. Simply observe the rising and falling of the abdomen or the touch of the air in or around the nostrils as you breathe in and out.

4. Open your eyes; let your gaze fall on your painting, drawing, or sculpture; and continue your breathing. Try slowly allowing the artwork to become the focus of your mind. Like *vipassana* meditation, try to stay with the image and your breathing, gently noting any sensations, thoughts, or distractions that come into your mind.

5. Try being present to your artwork for ten minutes at a time, gradually increasing to twenty minutes with practice. Take a few minutes after each sitting to write down what you remember about your experience, particularly any insights you experienced.

Being present often helps me to discover my visual work from a different perspective and, at the very least, is a calming, centering process with some of the same benefits as meditation.

WHEN NO ANSWER COMES

When I first began to make images from an authentic place within myself, I usually did not have an immediate explanation for the contents that emerged. In fact, sometimes I felt embarrassed in workshops or classes where people seemed to make art and know in great detail what their images meant to them. They were able to expound on each and every form, color, and symbol, relating them to the circumstances and events of their lives. I wondered if I had some serious blockage in my ability to make sense of my creations or to deny that which was painful or revealing.

Fortunately, I gradually realized that my process of receiving wisdom from my images had a different rhythm, one that allowed understanding to emerge slowly over time. I was impressed that the soul's palette intuitively respected my need to take in new information at a pace that was emotionally right for me. I also recognized that images often emerge well before words are possible, and, in some cases, as a preview of where I am headed in life well before I know it.

What do you do if nothing comes to mind, and you're feeling totally stumped or blocked? First, don't worry. It is not necessary to have an understanding of each image when you create it. Meanings often come about slowly, with some ideas appearing soon after the image is completed, and many others emerging with time. Don't expect to be able to immediately associate, amplify, or understand everything you draw, paint, or construct; just enjoy the process as well as the expectation that their messages to you will reveal themselves when the time is right. The wonder of the soul's palette is its compassion and sensitivity in expressing and illuminating self-knowledge at a pace that is attuned to your readiness to receive its wisdom.

Your images will undoubtedly have different meanings over time, as days, weeks, and even years pass. Don't think that your task is over once you have defined what an image means in a particular painting or drawing. Instead, that meaning may change, or the meaning that you have discovered may provide clues when you look at other artworks you have created. An image changes each time we attend to it because our connection to it is always re-created in that particular moment.

What is important is to keep an open mind, try to stay free of conclusions, and continue your exploration. Our artistic souls can live with and even enjoy not knowing for a while. The more we can hold off on judgment and openly explore what we encounter through images, the more we expand our own imagination's capacity to make new connections and find delight in the mystery.

Remember that the process of image making is just as important as finding meaning for your work. The process itself is a truly transformative part of any art-making experience. Above all else, keep enjoying creating. Making meaning will eventually fall into place if you stay with and continue to nourish your creative source.

WORKING ALONE OR TOGETHER

Working alone. Finding meaning for your images is a process you can enjoy on your own. All of the techniques and ways of making meaning described above are forms of transformational practice carried on in the safety of your own studio. Working alone is a good path to take if you feel you don't need or want to share your images and process with others. There is something wonderful about having art and imagination in your life just for yourself.

There are many moments in my own art making that I delight in keeping private, a gift that I give to myself. Many of my image journals are like secret diaries; I feel that part of their curative power for my soul is the boundary I maintain about sharing their contents and the process of their creation. I learned at one point in my life that I wished I had the opportunity to keep my images safe from those who were not sensitive to their meaning and sacredness. When I was studying art therapy in graduate school, as a student I recall being given little choice about sharing an image journal that we were required to keep as part of a course. Our assignment was to make images of our feelings about the class, what we were learning through drawings or paintings, and to write about our images, making associations about the contents and what they might mean. The assignment was immensely helpful to me in developing my personal visual language, and I still have those journals, now twenty years old.

The problem with that experience was one of safety. We were required to turn in our image journals every few weeks to the instructor so she could give us feedback on our creative work. Unfortunately, the instructor gave approval based on her own rules of creative expression and talked openly in class about the contents of our image journals. This felt invasive, and my creative source was suddenly influenced by the circumstance of pleasing an instructor who passed judgment and neglected safety in the experience of image making. My expressive work gradually felt contrived because it was being evaluated by someone else's standards and I had to guard my outpourings.

You may feel that your image making is confidential because it is a place where you can let loose and be uninhibited in your expression and experimentation. Is your image making for anyone to see or for your eyes only? It may be important for you to inform others who share your space—family, friends, or roommates—that for now your image work needs to remain private. Showing your creative work to others is part of the joy of self-expression, but only when you are ready to and feel supported and safe about doing so.

Working with a therapist. There are some benefits to working with another person as a witness to your process, particularly if that person is skilled in understanding how creativity helps and heals. Many people who consult an expressive or art therapist have already found their creative source on their own and have been using it for some time before they decide they want to work with another person. At some point an issue, feeling, circumstance, or image emerged that called to be shared or to simply hear someone else's reflection on their images.

At other times, we don't necessarily need reflection, advice, or wisdom; we need someone to create a holding space for us to create or process what we have created. In psychotherapy, a holding space is the environment the therapist creates with an individual in order to ensure a sense of safety, freedom, and respect. In art therapy, this goes beyond the therapist and includes the space where art is made and how it is witnessed, discussed, and amplified.

The benefit of sharing your images with a person who can support your creative process is that it can help you to deepen your understanding of the messages your creative source generates. This can be particularly important if you are going through a difficult life experience such as loss, trauma, or illness. We don't always need to go it alone; if you are in the midst of a rough time emotionally, look for someone who has skills in supporting your journey and can create a holding space for your creative process.

Working within a group. There may be times when it feels right to try art making within a group or community space or studio. Creating images within a group has a long tradition in most of the world's cultures. People have always gathered to create visual rituals, objects, and images to be used to honor or commemorate significant life experiences and to express themselves in the presence of family, friends, or communities.

Making art in the presence of others is different from making art alone. In a group your images can be seen by many and your stories can be heard by those you choose to tell. Being in a group can also be a challenge, especially if you feel easily distracted or are intimidated by working on your art while others are in the same room or space. Some groups have a facilitator, while others facilitate themselves. The benefit of a facilitator is that one person is responsible for the group for art making to take place and helps the group to receive, honor, and respond to the art created within the group.

It is worth taking the risk of entering a group setting because of the unique creative energy that exists only within the presence of others. Studio groups offer an energy that may inspire you to develop your work or may stimulate new ways of image making. Every time I work in the presence of others, I learn something that excites me to want to make more art. I also find that the energy that others bring to the space enlivens me and keeps me engaged through the atmosphere of creativity that is generated. Creating in the vicinity of other people who are also creating brings about a synergy that you will not find in your own studio working alone.

Making art with a group can be a powerful wellness practice. First, it requires that you commit yourself to participating over a period of time, perhaps months. As I indicated earlier, the commitment to regular practice is a positive force that imparts energy to our intentions for well-being. The group practice also offers benefits that only communal settings can provide, including social interaction, exchange of ideas and feelings, witnessing and support, and sharing the creative spark and passion for art making.

Finding a story and meaning for your creative work is an important part of its potential to heal, make whole, and create wellness. You can deepen the process by using art to care for yourself in all areas of your life, including body, mind, heart, and spirit. In the next several chapters you will learn ways to use your creative source for physical health, emotional peace, and spiritual well-being.

SEVEN

Images as a Path to Physical Well-Being

any cultures, both ancient and contempo rary, have embraced the power of mental images to produce positive changes in the body. Ancient Greeks and Romans actually believed that images moved through the blood, directly influencing physical functioning and emotions. Today, traditional cultures of North America such as the Navaho use sandpainting in rituals designed to enhance the mind's ability to rejuvenate and strengthen the body's inner resources to regenerate and heal. Modern medical practice now recognizes the power of images in the treatment of people of all ages, and arts medicine is a growing part of daily life in hospitals and clinics.

In this chapter you will learn how art as medicine can help you to manage illness, to reduce stress, and to heal. Your creativity can help you to cope with pain or other debilitating symptoms and identify deeper messages from the soul that may contribute to illness. Art making naturally taps your body's inner knowing and can be your doorway to deeper understanding of illness or trauma, conveying powerful messages about your physical being.

IMAGES AS MESSENGERS OF THE BODYMIND

There is clear evidence that mind and body are intricately connected and that our physical being naturally strives toward wellness and adaptability. This interplay between psychological and physical states is a unity referred to as the bodymind.

Body and mind reflect and influence each other with astonishing faithfulness. Our thoughts and feelings affect the health of our bodies and how we function from day to day. Science now recognizes that experiences like chronic depression may increase the risk of heart disease and other illnesses. Even simple experiences of anxiety or fright cause physical symptoms such as nausea, rapid heartbeats, or sweaty palms.

A young woman once came to see me with some drawings she had made in response to disturbing dreams she had had. The first drawing was of a rotting peach with black mold on it. In the dream she tried to clean the spot from the peach, but the more she cleaned, the darker the mold became. Her other drawings of dreams had a similar theme—a dark spot or marking on a plant or other living thing.

The dreams were so distressing that she intuitively felt something must be terribly wrong. Several months later a dark mole appeared on her forearm, and because of her dreams and drawings, she immediately had it evaluated. It was malignant melanoma, but owing to her urgency, surgery was performed in time to stop the cancer from spreading throughout her body.

While witnessing the soul's palette in others has convinced me that it often communicates the wisdom of the bodymind, my own firsthand experience made me a true believer. Many years ago, for the first time in my adult life I became suddenly ill with a variety of symptoms: swollen and painful joints, low-grade fevers, great fatigue, and general malaise. For a while I dismissed the symptoms as nothing serious and tried to forget about the pain, stiffness, and debilitation, thinking they would certainly go away with time. I invented reasons for my increasing fatigue, but each day I became worse until finally I could no longer deny that something was terribly wrong.

On one particularly bad day, I got out my sketchbook and made a drawing of a black figure that I remembered dreaming about during

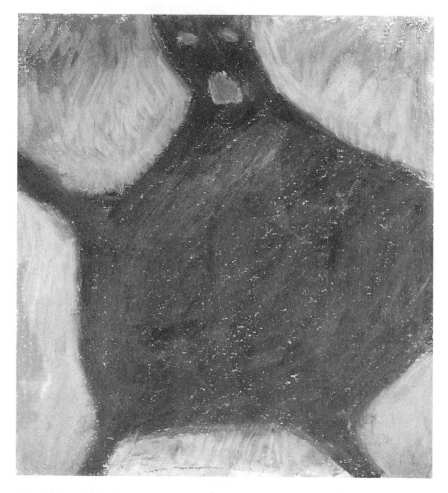

Black Spectre, dream drawing by the author.

the previous month. The image looked like a cellular being or maybe something alien from another world. The black figure had a chilling effect on me, and I became suddenly afraid that I was becoming disabled. For the first time I admitted to myself that I was exhausted, was less able to concentrate and remember, and was losing weight. Later that week, the more I tried to do, the more overwhelming my fatigue became and I retired to bed to sleep twelve hours or more a day. My head was constantly swimming with a relentless fever, my thoughts were disorganized, and my short-term memory was nonexistent. I felt like a victim of dementia and on some days worried that I might never be completely healthy again.

In the following months of going to internists, orthopedic specialists, and rheumatologists, I was given the diagnosis of either a chronic viral infection similar to chronic fatigue syndrome or an autoimmune illness. I was very ill for months, and all I could do was stay in bed. With no physical vitality, I decided to make the most of my waking hours, drawing in my sketchbook, recording the progress of my illness.

Messages from my body came not only through personal symbols such as the black, alien figure but also in my intuitive use of color. With great regularity I would begin to use red just before a bout of joint pain or the onset of a fever. A yellowish green appeared in my art whenever I was about to have digestive upsets; orange, a color I rarely used in my work before becoming ill, emerged during periods of intense fatigue. When things went wrong all over my body, black would come into my pictures, generally in the form of images that looked like cells or one-celled microscopic creatures. Although I never arrived at a clear explanation of these figures, I came to appreciate the consistency of the colors and forms that spontaneously appeared in my small sketches.

When the initial veil of illness began to lift after months of debilitating symptoms, my drawings suddenly took on a deeply metaphoric quality and contained many symbols of rebirth such as eggs or green, growing plants. My drawings also became larger—I went from 6-x-9 to 18-x-24-inch white paper almost overnight. This probably reflected my increased energy to some extent, but it also revealed the renewal and recovery my bodymind was experiencing. My dream world was also active in telling me about my pending recovery. During this time of increasing wellness, I dreamed that a hand that was holding me underwater suddenly released me and I buoyed upward to gasp at the air. It was easy to see that I was emerging from below the surface of life and back into the world.

Not every black image or dark spot is symbolic of cancer or illness, but our ability to create images in our imagination, in dreams,

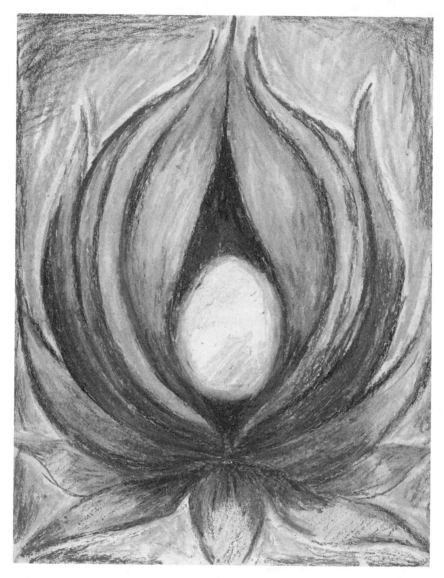

Rebirth, drawing of an image of recovery by the author.

or on paper can help us intuit messages from the bodymind. Images reflect the intelligence of the body and mind about the presence of wellness or illness, sometimes long before we even know we are sick.

DREAMS AS GUIDES TO THE BODYMIND

There is an Algonquin healing song that says:

> It was told to me in a dream
> That I should do this
> And I would recover.[1]

The belief that dream images can alert us to physical changes or signal impending illness has a long tradition dating back to at least the ancient Greeks. Hippocrates, father of modern medicine, noted that certain dream images predicted future illnesses. He also observed that dreams could confirm one's physical fitness, claiming that clear and vivid images of the sun, moon, and heavens, trees thriving and in bloom, and rivers flowing were all signs of excellent health. Galen, a second-century physician, believed that images found in dreams were a diagnostic tool and used information from his own dreams and those of his patients to prepare remedies and treatments. Tribal shamans have described learning the medicinal uses of specific plants through dreams and visions.

Medicine and psychology recognize the existence of "prodromal" dreams that diagnose disease or indicate early symptoms of illness. The woman who dreamed of spotted fruit had what could be called a prodromal dream; she felt that her dream images were powerful guides to pay attention to her body and well-being. My drawing of a black figure was likely prodromal, too; it appeared in advance of my worst symptoms of fatigue, fever, and malaise. Dreams and imagery have equally been associated with physical recovery, spontaneous healing, and health remedies.

Jung valued dreams for the intuitive messages they contained about appropriate treatments for physical conditions. He was once asked to interpret the following description of a dream, without being given any other information about the patient:

> Someone beside me kept asking me something about oiling some machinery. Milk was suggested as the best lubricant. Apparently I thought that oozy slime was preferable. Then, a pond was drained and amid the slime there were two extinct animals. One was a minute mastodon. I forgot what the other one was.[2]

Based on this dream, Jung correctly determined that the patient had a blockage of cerebrospinal fluid due to a tumor. While his rationale for the diagnosis was intuitive and based on his understanding of symbols, it is easy to understand that the dream conveyed a malfunction of some sort (in this case, a machine in need of a lubricant).

Author and editor Marc Ian Barasch had an experience with dreams that convinced him of their predictive power as well as their ability to change the course of a serious illness. In the midst of a successful career in his outer life, Barasch suddenly encountered an ominous turn in his dream world, which became vivid and emotionally jolting. In one dream an escaped murderer was chasing him with an ax to decapitate him, and in another, a figure symbolizing Death peered into his basement window, coolly casing his house. Many of the dreams had something to do with the neck—long needles stuck into his neck and a World War II bullet lodged in his neck. While he could make no immediate sense of these images, he found them deeply disturbing and unlike anything else he had ever experienced in his dream world. He was sure that something inside him had gone drastically wrong.

Finally, Barasch had a complete medical workup, and a tumor in his neck was discovered. At first, the doctor thought it was benign, but the nightmarish images of Barasch's dreams told the dreamer that it was serious. In a subsequent biopsy a cancerous malignancy was found. His dreams of danger, death, and necks had been frighteningly prophetic of his bodymind's wisdom. Barasch also dreamed of the doctor who would eventually do the surgery to remove his cancerous tumor. In the dream about having a bullet in his neck, a kindly Chinese surgeon removed it. Barasch's surgeon indeed turned out to be Chinese, leaving him to trust his dreams as much as X rays, CT scans,

and blood tests. In his wo
"take the pulse of the soul

Although some dreams
dreams that appear to be a
physical illness. Most of ι
prodromal but, in fact, c
Garfield, expert on dream
record of dreams that see
images are particularly v
quality to them different
dreams in this way may h
to health and well-being.

that result from psychologic
want to face. Images are
and, as such, have the
and to bring welln
Shaun McNi
that each ti
available
format
soul

ART AS MEDICINE FOR THE BODYMIND

Dreams are not the only important source of images that reflect physical health or illness. Your artistic creativity can also express symptoms,
the course of illness, and critical changes in health and well-being.
Imagery, either in the form of visualization or drawing, can actually
be predictive of the course of physical illnesses. Susan Bach, who spent
decades studying the artwork of seriously ill children, found common
images in their drawings that correspond to their illnesses and often
reveal healing or remission. For example, children who were in the last
stages of cancer and near death drew roads leading toward the upper
left quadrant of the paper or sketched butterflies, a symbol of transformation. Bernie Siegel anecdotally observes similar experiences in
his patients. When illness is difficult to describe with words, we may be
able to more accurately convey our physical symptoms through artistic creativity than through language.

Susceptibility to illness has often been linked with unresolved
emotional conflicts. While images can be a reflection of the bodymind,
dreams or self-created images of illness are not purely emotional messages
or something that you have been repressing. For example, heart disease is not simply a metaphor for a person's fear of opening his heart,
and cancer is not the repression of unexpressed anger or the inability
to nurture oneself. The body's wisdom is not just a set of symptoms

al dysfunction or a fear that one does not
loving messengers from the soul's palette
potential to remind us to take care of ourselves
ss and wholeness to both the body and the soul.
f observes that art offers medicine for the soul and
e we engage in art making, art's medicine becomes
o us. While the images we construct can communicate in-
on about the body's condition, what nurtures and heals the
in times of illness is the creative process of authentic and satis-
ying self-expression.

Finding your way to wellness through art making and imagination is a personal process, one that has many paths and possibilities. I
think that each of us has a capacity to cultivate an inner knowing
about our bodies through art expression and image work. Like the
woman who felt distressed about the spotted peach, you can tap your
creative source to enhance your understanding of the bodymind. Images can help you to literally see what your body is saying and whether
body, mind, and soul are out of balance. Taking the time to commune
with the body through image strengthens your understanding of your
physical self and hones your natural ability to intuit when something
goes wrong. In its simplest form, it can help you to pay attention to
physical messages you might otherwise overlook.

Image making is a powerful practice to enhance your sense of
well-being and wholeness, even in times of serious illness. Whether
you are physically ill or in good health, using your artistic creativity
to stimulate the flow of communication between body and mind is a
wellness practice. When undertaking any of the activities and practices in this book, please do not use them as a substitute for appropriate medical intervention. Rather, it is important to use your
creative source as a *complement* to medical treatment, as one part of
your overall wellness program.

DRAWING BREATH

James Joyce once wrote of a character, "Mr. Duffy lived a short distance from his body." Many of us are not aware of how our bodies feel

or react. Sometimes it is not until we are exhausted, develop chronic pain, or even become seriously ill that we gain awareness of how our bodies actually feel.

Becoming more aware of our breath is a simple activity that can help us reconnect with our feelings and bodily sense. The act of breathing is one of the most fundamental processes of life itself. In many sacred traditions, the breath is recognized as the source of vital energy for both body and mind. Yogis have demonstrated in scientific laboratories that it is possible to alter body temperature, heart rate, and metabolism through slowing the breathing. Transpersonal psychiatrist Stanislav Grof, in his research on consciousness, has demonstrated that breathing practices can create altered states, transcendence, and healing.

As children, we breathe fully, deeply, and freely; as adults, we often lose this simple skill because of stress and other factors. When we are frightened we may hold our breath, an action that often stops us from sensing or feeling our bodies. Many of us have acquired a habit of shallow breathing that physiologically actually increases our sensations of fear or anxiety.

"Drawing breath" is a way to get in touch with your breathing and life force. There is a basic meditation on the breath, practiced throughout the world, that I find even more effective for the bodymind when combined with drawing. Its purpose is to help you breathe from your belly rather than from your chest and to become conscious of your body's sensations, sense of balance, and centeredness.

1. Imagine that the bottoms of your feet are open and that energy from the earth can be received through them. With your eyes closed and your feet firmly on the ground, inhale slowly, visualizing the energy that you are bringing into your body from the earth. Consciously think about breathing into your belly rather than your chest. Exhale, watching the energy within you going back through your feet and into the earth. Repeat this for a few minutes. Try to think of the in-breath as strengthening and empowering you, and the out-breath as a force that cleanses and purifies you.

2. Stop, open your eyes, and slowly try drawing your inhalations and exhalations on paper. Let yourself intuitively make lines and shapes

across the paper and use colors that best represent the quality of your breathing. Keep breathing slowly and deeply into your abdomen, and keep making marks and images on the paper that reflect the movement of energies through your body. Continue this process for five to ten minutes or as long as you like and on as many sheets of paper as you like.

This exercise is very helpful in keeping you in touch with how you are breathing and develops a quiet awareness within. If you find this activity helpful, try some other experiments with your breathing:

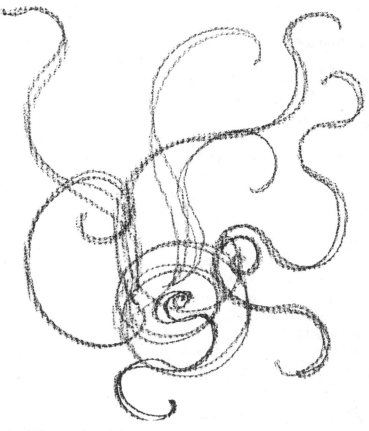

Example of "drawing breath."

◆ Again, imagine that the bottoms of your feet are open and that the earth's energy can be received through them. With your eyes closed and your feet firmly on the ground, inhale slowly, and this time imagine that that energy is a spiral. Imagine that this spiral of energy comes into your body in a counterclockwise direction and, on the exhalation, leaves in a clockwise direction. Continue this process for several minutes, stop, open your eyes, and continue your spiral breathing while drawing these energies on a large piece of paper.

◆ Practice the same breathing exercise, but while focusing on different areas of your body. Try breathing energy into your feet and legs, your pelvis, your stomach, your heart, your throat, and your head. At each area, take three to five complete in-breaths and out-breaths. Usually three breaths will help you to focus on a particular area, but continue breathing for a longer period of time into areas that need more attention. Experiment with visualization during this activity, and try to imagine the color of your breathing as it enters each area of your body. Try imagining different colors and be aware of which colors energize or calm you. Make a drawing of this experience, in the form of either a drawing of your body or any shapes, images, or colors that came to mind during your meditative breathing.

With regular practice for a few minutes a day, drawing breath can help you to increase your bodymind awareness, reduce stress, and teach you how to be in the moment, an experience of peace that nourishes your body and sense of well-being. Most of all, it teaches you to take your time and take inventory of your physical energy on a regular basis.

DRAWING ON BODY WISDOM

In working with people who are ill or have physical symptoms, I often suggest that they use their artistic creativity to learn their bodymind's language. Image making is a way of knowing our own inner rhythms and becoming more sensitive to our own body's cycles. Like dreams, our creative source can be a conduit to the signs and symbols of illness, debilitation, recovery, and healing.

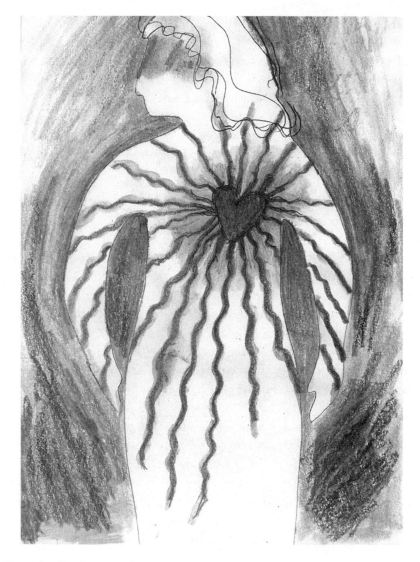

Example of body image drawing.

To tap your body's inner knowledge, try using an image of your own body as a starting point for image making. On a sheet of white paper or in your image journal, draw a silhouette of your body with a pencil or pen. Don't worry about proportions or appearance; just make an outline of your body, including a head, torso, hands and arms, and feet and legs. Intuitively color the inside of your body out-line with whatever colors, lines, shapes, or images that come to mind. Be spontaneous. If you feel the urge to color your feet purple or put spirals on your head, then do so. You can also draw outside the lines and add any colors, lines, or images around your body that you wish to include.

Put your image up on the wall or someplace where you can stand back and look at it. Think about what colors, lines, or images you in-cluded and where you placed them. Try inventing dialogues with these characteristics, as described in chapter 6, and write down these dialogues on paper or in your journal. Continue this exercise over the next month; usually, over time, you will begin to see patterns in your use of color, forms, and images. The images are reflective of your own personal visual logic and the language of your bodymind.

If you are currently struggling with illness or pain, try using this activity as a record of symptoms from day to day or week to week. For example, maybe today you have a headache and fatigue. What colors, shapes, and images describe these sensations? Again, use your imag-ination to draw and color intuitively, rather than getting caught up in concrete, realistic representations. Over time you may be able to identify cycles, seasons, or other time-related patterns of symptoms or illness.

Anna, a woman who came to see me for help with stress and de-pression, had an interesting experience using the body-outline activ-ity over the course of a month. She had a very stressful job in a public relations company and often felt exhausted from severe headaches that forced her to stay in bed for hours. Her bodymind's wisdom came through loud and clear in a series of body outlines that she col-ored over a couple of weeks. Anna realized that she put a lot of energy and time into coloring the area around her jawline and neck with bright red, orange, and fuchsia. She suddenly became aware of all the tension she stored in her jaw, especially when she had to present her ideas at meetings.

As it turned out, when she recognized this tension in her images, Anna also began to realize how much she felt silenced by some of her colleagues at work. Her intense emotional stress, along with the sen-sations in her jaw, went unrecognized until her creative source's own intuitive knowing became visible in her simple coloring. In subsequent sessions, we were able to take this process in a direction to help Anna develop her own art medicine on her body's behalf. She created a transformative image of clouds moving across her face and neck; this became a visual cue to remember to relax her jaw, thus eliminating most of her debilitating headaches.

Think of the body outline activity as a source of transformation. What colors, shapes, and images would be helpful in achieving wellness? In other words, rather than using the outline as a record of symptoms and sensations, use it imaginatively to create your own health-giving image of yourself. If you are having health problems or simply are experiencing physical symptoms as a result of stress, try making this activity into a regular practice by engaging in it three times a week for as long as it seems helpful.

If you find this activity beneficial or simply enjoyable, try making a life size body outline. Have a friend trace your body on a large sheet of craft paper, or simply create a life-size body outline of your own. Because this image is much bigger than the original body outline activity, you may find it more satisfying to use photographic images collected from magazines or brushes and paint to fill in the outline.

MAKING AN ART MEDICINE POUCH

Rituals and ritual objects have been used for centuries as a means to reduce illness and suffering and have been central to wellness practices in all of the world's cultures. Whether you are confronting the effects of illness or are just invested in continuing good health, you may find that adding rituals and ritual objects is soothing and healing to your bodymind.

When I was ill, I felt vulnerable and afraid, especially when I was not getting well and I had to face continual tests and doctor visits that often resulted in more bad news. Life became awfully lonely while I sat in a waiting room for several hours to see a specialist or in a cold hallway to get an X ray or another blood draw. Sometimes my husband or a friend would sit with me, but I felt I needed some other source of support to see me through the darker days.

A friend, a member of the local Paiute tribe, told me about a healing ceremony she had witnessed many times, conducted by a medicine man. She carried a pouch that contained objects and herbs that were used to cure various illnesses and conditions. She also told me that newborn children in her tribe were given a pouch with important objects that family members contributed to help and protect the child later in life.

Inspired by her account, I decided to make myself a bag with items in it that I felt would help me through the days of debilitation I faced. I fashioned it out of some leather scraps, fabric, and feathers and added a strap so that I could wear it as well as carry it. I began to gradually add objects that held positive meaning for me—an oak leaf from my birthplace in Connecticut, a postcard of a reindeer my husband sent me from a trip to Norway, an owl's feather found on a hike, a poem by Rumi that a friend sent, a sprig of lavender, and some small crystal stones. These were my personal ritual objects, like the magic items in the Paiute medicine man's bag.

I began to carry the pouch on doctor appointments or anytime I felt the need to have some wellness symbols with me. Sometimes I would just think about the objects inside the pouch, and on other occasions I would take out some of the items and meditate about their meaning or simply enjoy them as images. To my surprise, my art medicine pouch turned out to be a conversation piece that attracted questions from the technicians, nurses, and fellow patients. Part of its magic was all the interactions that it stimulated when someone asked about it or wanted me to reveal its contents. On occasion, someone would give me something to add to the pouch or I would add a card with a loving message recently sent by a friend. The more I carried the pouch, the more good wishes and support from others I received.

I realize now that the pouch and its magic contents simply tapped the courage that I possessed deep within me but had lost during a time of severe stress. We all are afraid when our lives are threatened with disability, extended illness, and the possibility of death. At such a time, a bit of ritual and a little placebo effect (the power of belief in a treatment or medicine) can really help.

You can make your own art medicine pouch out of felt or fabric, either sewing or gluing the edges together to form a pouch or bag.

Decorate the outside with feathers, beads, or sequins. In adding images or other objects to your pouch, think about what items make you feel safe, remind you of someone or something dear to you, or simply give you sensory pleasure. We all have treasured objects, photos, cards, or quotations that hold special meaning for us; these are the perfect talismans to include in the pouch. You may also want to create several small collages or drawings that represent any of the following:

- something that gives you happiness
- something that was difficult in life that you were able to overcome
- someone or somewhere that makes you feel safe

Since the time I was ill, I have made a series of art-medicine pouches that sit on my desk, in the studio, and by my bedside; sometimes I take one along with me on a trip. I think it is a form of preventive art-medicine to have these containers close by while I am away from home and to look at images and objects that remind me of experiences and qualities that give me strength and inner peace.

TRANSFORMATIONAL WELLNESS PRACTICES

Try any of the following ideas to reduce stress or symptoms and to enhance your sense of wellness through regular practice.

Shift your perceptions. How you relate to pain and physical discomfort has a lot to do with your state of mind. When I had painful joints, the more I tried to ignore the pain, the more noticeable it became. One day I thought, "Well, if I can't get away from this pain, I may as well make something out it." I started to do the opposite of what I was trying to do—ignore the pain—and instead focused on the sensations, doodling in my sketchbook whatever came to mind. Before I knew it, an hour had passed and I had been so lost in my drawing that my painful joints, even the ones in my hands, were not an issue.

Art making can help to shift your perceptions of symptoms and sometimes even transform them. Consider artistic expression as a way to change your beliefs, try out new ways of being with your illness or symptoms, or reconnect with "remembered wellness" from a time when you were physically healthy. Use your creative source anytime you need to simply have some time away from your medical condition or symptoms. Seeing yourself as an artist can become a natural replacement for seeing yourself solely as a patient with a particular diagnosis or illness.

Assess your wellness resources. For many years, Bernie Siegel asked his patients to do simple drawings addressing two questions: What do you think about your illness, and what do you think about treatment? He chose these questions because they are related to the ability to achieve well-being no matter what the disease or prognosis. Making images of your illness and your treatment will help you to understand how you feel about both your physical well-being and the medical interventions that are being prescribed to help make you well.

Tap your dreams for their knowledge of the bodymind and your own intuition about your body and medical treatments. Create an image journal based on your dreams, recording either images or sensations you remember about your dreams in color, line, and shapes. If you decide to make a dream image journal, be sure to work on it as soon as you awaken each morning. Dream images are often fleeting, and we tend to forget details as the day passes. Include any written descriptions along with your images in order to help you remember as much as possible about the content and emotional qualities of your dreams and their relationship to your bodymind.

Create a picture of health. If you are suffering from a health problem or symptom, use your imagination to help you create a picture of health, an intention for future well-being. To enliven your mental ability to imagine healing or recovery, try making a collage that depicts the various aspects of your intention. If, for example, your intention is to reduce chronic pain, collect pictures from magazines that represent an environment that decreases your symptom. You may be drawn to pictures of warmth such as the sun or the beach if that helps your pain, or to places in nature that help you to relax and reduce stress. The more vivid and colorful the images are, the better.

To personalize your intention, include a photo of yourself in the center of your collage. Glue all the images on a large piece of paper or cardboard. Hang your picture of health in a place where you will see it each day. You may also tape the images around the perimeter of a mirror that you look into each day. What is important is that you experience these images daily, even if only for a few moments. Your imagination will take in their positive messages for well-being and incorporate your intentions for renewed or increased health in the here and now.

Seeing images that give you pleasure on a regular basis is a wellness-inducing practice and enhances your internal resources to heal. It may also be a way to help you manage symptoms that are preventing you from doing things you wish to do. An artist friend was recently diagnosed with the first stages of emphysema, a condition that causes severe breathing difficulties and physical and emotional distress. He believed that imagery might alleviate the sensations of tightness and respiratory distress he was experiencing from time to time. Since he spent a large portion of his day in his studio, he decided to try surrounding himself with images of wide-open spaces, the sky, and clouds in the form of photographs and his own paintings on the walls and ceilings. These images were his personal metaphor for being able to breathe deeply, relax, and feel healthy. Now, every time he feels constriction or breathing problems, he meditates on the imagery around his studio and finds that he feels less debilitated by his condition.

Paint or draw your emotional responses to illness. If you sense that your illness has an emotional basis, you may want to try to depict how you feel about your symptoms or condition. When I was very ill, I found that drawing my anger or anxieties about my pain, fever, and debilitation helped to reduce symptoms in several ways. First, it provided an emotional release and a place to express responses that I could not articulate with words. On a deeper level, it helped to clear the anger, sadness, and fears I had about my symptoms and to regain some energy and stamina.

Witness, reflect on, or dialogue with your images as much as you feel you need to. Writing about my images when I was ill was often as helpful as the actual making of them. Writing helped me to articulate to myself what I was experiencing, gradually release my sense of loss, and go on with life. I started to bring my image journal to medical appointments because it helped me to communicate my more confusing symptoms to my doctor and to recall the cycle of pain or fever. Sometimes it was helpful to reflect on my images with another as a witness—a therapist or supportive friend. Think about what feels right for you in terms of sharing your images with others, especially if you feel alone or isolated by your illness or symptoms.

USING YOUR MIND'S EYE

At times during my illness, I did not always have the physical energy or mental stamina to even make a simple drawing in my sketchbook. If you are debilitated, in extreme pain, or extremely fatigued, it may not be possible for you to draw or paint. Fortunately, you still have a very powerful wellness tool at your disposal—your imagination. Your imagination—the mind's eye—has a wonderful ability to see the past, present, and future simultaneously. In your imagination the future is happening right now and when you form a mental image of a goal or intention for the future, your imagination thinks it is real and present. Your mind's capacity to use images to transcend the here and now can help you to actualize goals and intentions in each and every part of your life, including health and well-being.

There are several simple practices you can use to enhance your sense of well-being through mental visualization. Each should be preceded by taking some time to fully relax your body and mind through progressive muscle relaxation, the breathing exercise described earlier in this chapter, or a short meditation. These practices work best when used on a regular basis and are more effective when repeated at least twice a day for ten to twenty minutes. Try using one or more of them just prior to falling asleep. Tapping the imagination with the intent to heal works best at bedtime because you are usually already in a relaxed state at that time of the day.

Use color to soothe your symptom. Form a mental picture of your favorite colors, and imagine those colors in the form of a beam of light. In your imagination, direct the beam of light to the areas where you need relief. For example, if you have back pain, imagine a source of colored light filling and soothing that part of your body. If you have trouble visualizing your favorite colors, imagine a white or golden light pouring through your body. You can also try a warm color (such as red) or a cool color (such as blue) to warm or cool the area of your body. Because color is a personal preference, experiment with this practice and decide which colors work best for you.

Imagine an outside source of healing. Try mentally picturing the part of the body that needs attention (such as your head, if your have a headache). Think of what that area of your body needs, such as warmth, coolness, or relief of tension. Now try to imagine what might provide that relief, such as sunlight, gentle water, or healing hands. For example, a person suffering from shoulder pain might try visualizing warm sunlight bathing and penetrating that part of the body. In your mind's eye, see the source of relief coming to your injured or ill body part, imagining it soothing and alleviating your symptoms.

Create a positive image of health or recovery. Try imagining yourself in optimal condition, seeing yourself engaged in a favorite activity or sport and participating without pain, discomfort, or worry. Visualize yourself as symptom-free, active, energetic, and joyful. What things give you pleasure and vitality in life? Try to see yourself in situations, activities, or experiences that give you happiness, energize you, or inspire you.

To increase the health-giving benefits of these practices, include some form of art making as part of the experience when you can or if it feels helpful. For example, after visualizing an outside source of healing, make a drawing of that source or paint any sensations that you imagined or felt during your practice. Or, before imagining yourself in optimal health, meditate on a photograph of yourself taken when you felt energized or free of pain. Connecting images to your visualization experiences will reinforce your imagination's powers and intention to enhance well-being and deepen your ability to use imagery to relieve or heal symptoms.

Allow yourself to notice which of these activities and practices is useful for you and which seem irrelevant. You may find that some activities do not appeal to you now but become important in a few weeks or months.

The soul's palette contains an incredible source of medicine, one that can serve you in times of illness or support your health maintenance program along with nutrition, exercise, and other wellness practices. But art's healing powers extend beyond the bodymind. In the next chapter, you will experience how your artistic creativity can revitalize your emotions, repair a broken heart, and restore you in times of loss or grief.

EIGHT

rt as Reparation
and Restoration

believe our ability to make symbols and images is, in
part, a reaction to our own suffering and the suffering
of others. In times of crisis, mourning, grief, and loss,
artistic expression helps us to convey and cope with powerful emotions,
to repair and transform feelings, and eventually to restore wholeness.

Emotional crisis is a potentially transformative experience, unveil-
ing a window through which illumination and knowledge can enter
our being. Creativity and imagination are often expanded during times
of trauma or loss. Your artistic creativity can open your heart and mobilize your natural capacity to heal painful experiences and feelings.
Art is a way of knowing your feelings on a deeper level; acknowledging, discharging, and reworking them; and seeing them in perspective. At the same time, the creative process can help you to shift away
from emotional stress in your life and awaken to experiences other
than suffering. Art has a power to pull us out of disappointment, confusion, or sadness. It is a way through pain and eventually out of it.

In this chapter you will learn why it is important to use images to
self-soothe and create positive sensations during times of stress. You
will learn why images can help you to find relief from crisis or pain.
Creative activities in this chapter will help you learn to express yourself from the heart and begin using art as a way to transform emotions.

We are all familiar with the stressful effects of holding on to anger, anxiety, or grief; unexpressed, these feelings can have harmful effects on the body, including severe disorders such as heart disease, chronic pain, or immune dysfunction. While no one is exempt from painful feelings, your creative resources and imagination are powerful and easily accessible tools for transforming and healing your emotions. This chapter will tell you how the very act of putting pencil to paper helps you allow feelings to surface and achieve greater emotional balance.

THE HEART OF THE SOUL'S PALETTE

One of the most impressive aspects of the soul's palette is its potential to achieve and restore emotional equilibrium. Carl Jung realized early in his work with patients and his own personal explorations that art expression and images found in dreams could be helpful in recovery from trauma and emotional distress. He often drew, painted, or made objects and constructions at times of emotional turmoil or personal crisis. Jung recognized his expression as more than mere recreation and believed that it helped him find insight into his struggles. In his memoirs, *Memories, Dreams, Reflections*, Jung describes an experience when he was ten years old that helped him overcome personal stress:

> I had in those days a yellow, varnished pencil case of the kind commonly used by primary school pupils, with a little lock and the customary ruler. At one end of the ruler I carved a little mannequin, about two inches long, with a frock coat, top hat, and shiny black boots. I colored him with black ink, sawed him off the ruler, and put him in the pencil case, where I made him a little bed. . . . This was all a great secret. Secretly I took the case to the forbidden attic at the top of the house . . . and hid it with great satisfaction on one of the beams under the roof. . . . I felt safe, and the tormenting sense of being at odds with myself was gone.[1]

For me, the emotionally healing qualities of art expression have taken many forms: paint and clay have contained ranting, crying, anger, hurt, and resentment. Art making is a companion that I don't have to worry about insulting or infuriating. On occasion, drawing has helped me to tell the story of a loss or death, or a photocollage might become a visual tribute to someone who has inspired me. In all instances, my creative source has been a natural pathway to help me open up by making my feelings visible through image.

Sharing powerful or disturbing feelings is now recognized as important to overall physical well-being. Artistic self-expression can help you explore, release, and understand the source of emotional distress, ameliorate trauma, and repair and resolve conflicts. Steve Nachmanovich suggests that art making is one of the best forms of psychotherapy available. I don't think he is necessarily suggesting that image making replaces the help of a professional. But your creative source has a low risk factor, psychically and financially, and can provide you with gentle, safe help. I believe we have a built-in, self-protective mechanism that prevents us from confronting emotions that we are not yet strong enough to feel and experience. This simply means that when we are not ready to draw or paint what is inside us, the worst that can happen is nothing emerges and we put down the brush or pencil for a while. Your inner artist reveals only as much of yourself as you are ready to see and understand.

TAPPING YOUR EMOTIONAL SHORTHAND

The writer Erica Jong once called imagery a kind of "emotional shorthand." I understand this to mean that while we may use paragraphs of prose to describe an emotional experience or event, images allow us to communicate directly and authentically. Art expression, imagination, and dreams are forms of emotional shorthand that help reconnect heart to body, mind, and soul during times of despair, confusion, and stress. If we experience severe emotional trauma, chronic stress, or loss and grief, we sometimes lose our verbal abilities to express our feelings. Many times the first step on the path back to accessing what is in our heart is through image work such as the following simple activities:

Explore your color vocabulary. Color is the underlying wisdom of your emotional shorthand. It reflects your thoughts, perceptions, and physical sensations but is most often associated with feelings. The colors you use in art, your home, your clothes, and your environment can help you to deepen your understanding of your emotional self.

Noting and comparing the colors you use to express your feelings through images can help you to understand how color reflects your emotional self. When people begin to explore feelings through art, either spontaneously or through keeping a visual feelings journal, they often naturally wonder about color and how it relates to emotions. As you work with the exercises in this book, you will begin to see that you have preferences for certain colors or that your use of color changes over time. While colors do often relate to how you feel, it is difficult to assign a specific meaning to any one color in your work. Many colors are associated with a variety of feelings, ideas, and connotations; some of these can be ambiguous or even contradictory. For example, while we associate red with love and passion, we also think of it as representing anger. When working with color, look for your own meanings and preferences.

Ask yourself the following questions about color in your images:

- How do I use color in my images to express emotion?

- Do certain colors have specific meanings for me?

- What colors have I used the most? Do any colors predominate?

- Do I like to use particular combinations, such as black and white; earthy, golden colors; pastels; deep, dark tones; hues found in nature?

Work with color spontaneously, but also try limiting your range of colors. With paint, oil pastels, or collage, try any or all of the following:

◆ Create an image with only your favorite colors; use colors that you like to wear or have around you in your environment.

◆ Create images using limited color ranges such as warm colors (reds, oranges, and yellows), cool colors (blues, blue-greens, lavender), colors of nature (browns, golden tones, greens), and simple black, white, and gray tones.

◆ How about the colors you never use? Perhaps these colors are not favorites or are simply colors you overlook in image making. Try making an image using only the rejected colors in your oil pastel set, tempera paints, or collage box.

As you work with color, realize that your use and preferences will change over time. For example, in drawing with oil pastels you will naturally begin to experiment with blending colors, learning more ways to make colors and to express yourself with new colors. As you experiment with color through various materials, your meanings and preferences for color will evolve and your emotional experiences of color will deepen.

Keep a feelings journal. Make a series of quick sketches with oil pastels, using color as your emotional shorthand to represent the feelings you are experiencing. In order to get the most from this activity, commit to it as a practice for at least a month, making a drawing several times each week. Try drawing from how your body senses the feeling rather than what your rational mind tells you about your emotional state. For example, if you are anxious, try to locate where that feeling is in your body and express that sensation on paper with color, line, and shape. Stay with your physical senses about feelings and be intuitive and spontaneous with your color choices.

Use emotion as a way to enter the art process. As a fluid medium, paint lends itself well to communicating emotion. To help you explore, express, and transform your feelings, create a series of small paintings of feelings. Prepare several surfaces such as watercolor paper, cardboard, or mat board with gesso; 11 x 14 inches is a good size to begin with. Using acrylic or tempera paints, choose colors that represent your mood, or simply paint spontaneously.

Create from movement in your body rather than your fingers. Perhaps your body feels tightly knotted into a ball or stretched out in all directions. Think about how you feel and how that could be expressed in lines or gestures across the surface, and see what develops. As with the scribble exercises in chapter 5, it is important to relax and find your own way of making images with paint. If you feel constrained or tense, try using your nondominant hand to paint, or use the ink-scribble

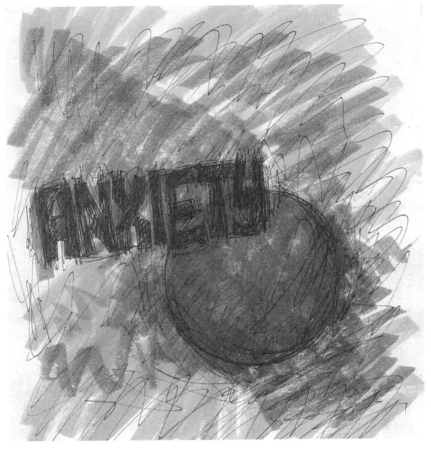

Image from a "feelings" journal.

technique to create lines and forms, filling them in with color or adding details with paint to create images.

Create for the joy of it. The soul's palette is about making art as you like, without concern for how it will be judged. Don't worry about being realistic or perfect; just paint or draw from what is inside you. If you are working from nature, try using colors that represent how you feel about trees, water, earth, and sky, rather than trying to duplicate the colors you see in front of you. Perhaps the sky is blue, but it feels warm or sultry to you; think about what color represents that feeling and what lines, forms, or shapes convey that idea. Use all the colors that give you joy, pleasure, a sense of renewal, and inspiration.

ACKNOWLEDGING THE HEART'S NEED TO HEAL

In Western culture, emotional strength is linked to endurance; when we experience a trauma or loss, we are urged to "get on with our lives" as quickly as possible. We carry on with a stiff upper lip, and those around us may even admire us for our apparent well-being. The problem comes when trauma or loss continue to be unexpressed and the effects become entrenched and chronic.

I have worked with people who are traumatized by life's most profound experiences: losses of loved ones through homicide or accidents, witnesses to violent crimes and school shootings, and survivors of cancer or other life-threatening illnesses. In the weeks of completing this book, I met with individuals who survived the terrorist attacks on the World Trade Center as well as those who were less directly affected but still emotionally shaken by the plane crashes, loss of life, and threats of biological warfare. Each person faced the difficult task of repairing and making whole a heart broken because of severe grief or nightmarish memories of events that rock the depths of the soul.

Research shows us that traumatic experiences in particular can become encoded in your mind in the form of images. That is, when you experience traumatic events, your mind captures them like a camera taking a photograph. However, these remembered images are not always accurate, and sometimes trauma can distort our memories of an event. The images you encode may be visual and may include a heightened sense of detail in the form of feelings, perceptions, and sensations. While you believe you have a literal and accurate recollection of what happened, mixed into this image are the emotions and sensations you experienced at the time of the trauma or crisis. Although memory may be distorted, the process of calling forth images after a trauma is still important to recovery and healing.

When we have been severely traumatized, memories may first reemerge in the form of images—dreams, visions, flashbacks, and visual fragments. Jean, whose story I told in chapter 1, is a good example of art's self-protective mechanism. Her images were like an early warning system that something was terribly wrong. They served as a safety valve to begin the process of releasing years of emotional pain and repairing a deeply wounded soul. Jean's creative source emerged before words and stories were available to her to explain their meaning.

Your artistic creativity can provide a way to express what is locked inside you, guiding traumatic images to consciousness in a less threatening way. Sometimes you simply need a tonic for your emotional self when you feel off balance or under stress. When a mood or problem appears as an image through a dream or art, you not only can begin to understand it more clearly and deeply but also can access all that is contained within it.

USING ART AND IMAGINATION TO CARE FOR THE HEART

There are a variety of ways to use art and imagination to recover from trauma, loss, or grief, or simply as a tonic for your emotional self when you feel stressed.

Self-Soothing Image Book

When we experience a serious trauma or loss, we often find ourselves avoiding sensory stimuli, particularly those which remind us of the event. Unfortunately, in the process of closing ourselves to such influences, we may also deprive ourselves of stimuli that could be soothing and healing. Images are a simple way to move yourself from a stressful state to one of calm or to give yourself a relaxation break.

I have created image journals over the years that I consider my self-soothing image books. One is a book of color swatches and pictures of interiors of homes that I enjoy. I originally created the book to collect design and paint color ideas for our home, but like most people, I never got around to most of the ideas I planned. Now I just keep gathering color swatches at the local home improvement store and magazines clippings of wonderful rooms and gardens. The book gives me pleasure when I flip through the pages and is filled with dreams and future plans for projects. Instead of feeling guilty or regretful that I never followed through on these redecorating projects, I feel good because I know I am treating myself to a health-giving break.

I also created a book with a theme of leaves picked up on all my travels and in my own backyard. I may press actual leaves and glue them onto the pages, or else I trace or draw interesting leaves, trees, and roots. I still have another fifty pages to fill, and like the book of interior design ideas, I visit it every so often just for the pleasure of looking at its contents.

By simply witnessing the materials in your collage box, you may find yourself attracted and soothed by certain images and materials more than others. Put aside these images, colors, and textures, and consider why and how they soothe your emotional self. Use these as the inspiration for a sensory image book and create a series of mini-collages using the images. If you don't have a journal to devote to this activity, try creating a simple handmade book with at least ten sheets of white paper or any other colored paper of the same size.

To inspire your first self-soothing book, make a quick list of sensory experiences that are pleasant for you. Think about any of the following:

- Environments or nature
- Sounds or music
- Tastes or scents
- Tactile sensations or textures
- A particular experience or event where you felt happy, content, or peaceful

Look through magazines and other collage materials for examples of images that represent the pleasant and soothing sensory experiences you listed. Cut out as many images as you find self-soothing. Try arranging your images into compositions or categorize them by type (outdoors, textures, animals, interiors, people). If you are using a series of loose pages, collate the pages by hole-punching them and placing them in a binder, take them to a copy shop and ask for a spiral binding, or gather the pages together with string or staples.

Take some time after you have completed the project to jot down some notes on a separate piece of paper:

◆ Describe your general thoughts and feelings while selecting materials for the book.

◆ Which sensory images did you favor over others?

◆ Look through the book and select an image or page that is particularly pleasant or soothing. Take a minute to focus on this image and enter into the sensory aspects of this picture. What do you experience when looking at that image or page?

If you continually feel stressed or are suffering from a serious trauma or loss, use your sensory image book as an ongoing practice. Consider creating a special collection of images that give you pleasure, and arrange and glue them on a large piece of cardboard. Put it in a simple frame and hang it where you can see your images on a regular basis.

Create a Healing Garden

At a wellness community in my area—a program where cancer patients receive support and education—there is what is called a "healing garden" on the grounds. There are several flagstone paths, colorful rocks, stone sculptures, and numerous plants, some of which are herbs known as natural remedies and tonics. On many occasions I have witnessed the powerful effects of the landscape design and sculptures on visitors who come to walk through or sit in the garden. Often, people who are friends of a cancer patient or a family member in the midst of struggling with grief over the death of a spouse or child comes to meditate or to simply enjoy the relaxing effects of natural surroundings.

Being in the presence of nature can have a positive effect on your emotional state. Whether a favorite beach or an aesthetically designed garden, nature gives our bodies and minds a boost during time of stress or emotional strain. It is now known that hospital patients recover more quickly from surgery or other treatments if they have a room with a view of nature. It seems that the images of the natural world hold powerful medicine that accelerates a sense of well-being and health.[2]

Try creating a healing environment of your own. It does not have to be grandiose; look around for a patch of land or a window box that can become your healing garden. My husband and I have been lucky to always have a view of a flower or vegetable garden from our bedroom window. While your nature images may be in an outdoor setting, in colder climates an indoor composition may be more useful. Consider ways you can bring nature indoors. Perhaps a well-arranged group of potted plants or interesting rocks, seedpods, shells, and a box with beach sand or soil can be your inspiration. Think of giving yourself a bouquet of flowers once or twice a month to add something alive and colorful to your indoor healing garden.

Make a Safe Box

Recently, a friend's grandchild was going through an emotionally difficult time after the death of a classmate due to cancer. While the ten-year-old understood what had happened to his classmate, the experience haunted him for several weeks to the point of his having nightmares and repetitive thoughts about the death. The grandmother wisely came up with a creative solution. One afternoon they decorated an old shoebox together, and the grandson made pictures of his upsetting feelings to place in the box. While he could take out the drawings anytime he wanted to think about his friend, he was literally and visually able to "put a lid on things" by closing the upsetting pictures into the box. The box honored and held his feelings, while keeping them from intruding on his sleep and thoughts.

We sometimes need a place where we can put away our feelings, if only for a few hours. If you find yourself obsessed or controlled by powerful emotions, create a symbolic place to keep those emotions contained. A simple cardboard box or large mailing envelope can be the container for an emotional experience that you are not quite ready to leave behind but wish to take a rest from now and then. Try to find a container that has a lid or a way to close it so that its contents cannot be seen. Decorate the container any way you wish.

Create images of your feelings, collect photos of a lost loved one, or gather any material that brings the emotional experience forward. Place these in your safe box and allow it to become the container for these feelings and experiences whether they be pain, sorrow, anger, or worry. If you find this activity helpful, use it as a transformational practice by making it an ongoing holding space for any new feelings that arise. Know that it will take some time and practice to appreciate your safe box as a container that will allow you some distance from exhausting feelings. Make a ritual of taking it out and putting it away to strengthen your imagination's power to help you find closure on stressful emotions you are experiencing.

Pocket Shrines

I learned about pocket shrines from a homeless street artist who was selling ornately decorated matchboxes at an outdoor market. He told me that they were magic boxes that represented people he had met on the streets as well as the events of his life. Because they were small, they could be carried in a pocket so that one could take the magic along on one's travels. Some had small photographs of individuals in them and others were simply painted or collaged with colorful papers and found objects. Since I was going through my "black bird" period at the time, I bought a matchbook that was embellished with a raven image and contained a black feather and a piece of coal inside.

An ordinary set of objects becomes a shrine when it is arranged and given special significance. Anything displayed or arranged with reverence or evoking mystery can become a shrine. Shrine making is a form of art making that reflects the human urge to assemble and arrange things in a meaningful way. It underscores our proclivity to use imagination to imbue objects with power for the purpose of wellness and stability.

Shrines have typically been created to commemorate and facilitate the process of grieving. Home altars are a popular tradition in Mexico,

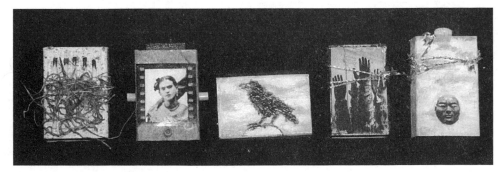

Matchbox "pocket shrines" by the author.

especially for the holiday known as the Mexican Day of the Dead (November 2, All Souls' Day), when the departed are honored by shrines that combine holy images (often the Virgin of Guadalupe), along with personal photographs, favorite foods, flowers, and other objects.

Since the time I met the street artist, I have made a pocket shrine or two every year, sometimes for no specific reason, and other times to commemorate a person. I have created several to honor a friend or family member or say good-bye to a lost loved one. Sometimes I have made one to symbolically contain a little magic or miracle, like a portable miniature Lourdes. It is enjoyable to work in a small format that you can hold in the palm of your hand. These shrines often seem very precious and special for this reason, and I find them comforting to have in my pocket or purse when I am feeling blue, afraid, or anxious.

For this activity you will need a small container such as a cardboard or plastic box or a matchbox. What is particularly nice about matchboxes is the way they slide open to reveal an inside compartment. You can decorate your box any way you wish, but consider the following ideas:

◆ If you are making a box to honor or remember someone, use a small photo of the significant other as either the outer or the inner image for your shrine. An inspiring teacher or other guide or mentor might be a good subject for such a shrine.

◆ Is there a special quote from an artist, philosopher, or spiritual mentor that you are inspired by? Write it out on a small piece of paper and make that the inner center of your box, decorating the rest of the box based on this source of inspiration.

◆ Put little treasures in your box—a pearl or crystal, a bird feather, a patch of animal fur, a small shell, or a trinket.

◆ Use paint, collage, and other embellishments to decorate your box.

The point is to create your own little piece of magic that you can carry with you in your pocket, handbag, or purse. Carry it with you for a month and observe how its images and contents serve you. If you find yourself in a stressful situation, hold or look at your pocket shrine and notice what happens. Over time you may find that you discover a sense of connection and peacefulness when you experience the images or objects in your shrine and the qualities they convey to you.

Drawing with Loving-kindness Meditation

Awakening your heart through meditation, affirmations, or acts of service not only heals your relationships with others but also nurtures your own emotional wounds. I believe that art making combined with meditation can help us to open to these healing influences. Before I do artwork or before entering a therapeutic session with an individual or group, I sometimes do *metta* meditation, the Buddhist practice of loving-kindness, which involves focusing on a series of phrases that help develop our natural heart qualities.

Loving-kindness means wishing for the happiness of others; it goes hand in hand with compassion, another important heart quality, which Buddhists define as wishing that others should be free from suffering. Tibet's Dalai Lama has been a model of these two virtues in our time. He has expressed his attitude of loving-kindness and compassion for the Chinese people, even though China invaded his homeland of Tibet in 1949 and forced the Dalai Lama into exile in India in 1959. The Dalai Lama knows that both hatred and loving-kindness have powerful but different effects on our hearts. Hatred only prolongs suffering, while compassion for those who may have harmed us frees us to enjoy living.

Before beginning the meditation, let your body relax and your mind become quiet, so that you can receive whatever emerges with friendliness and affection.

While there are many different phrases one can use in *metta* meditation, I like Jack Kornfield's from *A Path with Heart*:

> May I be filled with loving-kindness.
> May I be well.
> May I be peaceful and at ease.
> May I be happy.

You begin with yourself as the focus of *metta* meditation because without loving-kindness toward yourself, it is difficult to extend it to others. Kornfield suggests that as you say the phrases to yourself, picture yourself as a young and beloved child, or sense yourself as you are now, held in the heart of loving-kindness.

When you feel comfortable with yourself as a focus, try to gradually expand your loving-kindness to others. Picture someone who has taken care of you, reciting the same phrases, "May she/he be filled with loving-kindness," and so on. As your loving-kindness develops for this person, you can include others: friends, neighbors, animals, people in your city, eventually envisioning the whole world and all beings. With practice, you will find that you can include many beings in your meditation.

I have improvised the following affirmation as part of my meditation:

> Making art cares for my emotional self
> and by doing so,
> I am more compassionate to those around me.

I have learned over the years that I am a much more loving and generous person when I make art on a regular basis. Because art nourishes my soul, I have more to give to others when I am in touch with my creative source. Using this affirmation reinforces the idea that art making takes care of me while, at the same time, it deepens my ability to care for those around me.

It takes practice to develop genuine loving-kindness, and it takes even more practice to sustain it. But even after the first few times, this practice increases a sense of self-care, particularly for the emotional wounds within. I find that it puts me at peace when I feel the need to use art to address personal pain or suffering. It allows images to flow from my inner source of compassion and kindness and makes these blessings available to others. Through the meditation, my creative source is given the message that art making is a form of emotional self-care for heart and soul.

A Gratitude Scroll: Awakening the Heart to Thankfulness

Sometimes to heal a broken or troubled heart, we need to go outside of ourselves rather than focus only on what's inside. Like most people,

I have had my share of depression, anxiety, and stress. After one particularly stressful period, I decided to take a census of what was good in my life and see where that led my creative source. What came to mind was an image of a scroll, a kind of roll call of all that I experienced that gave me a feeling of gratitude. I started out with a long piece of paper and began to take an inventory of life's current assets: a loving relationship with my husband, the companionship of two cats, our health, our home, our garden, plenty of food, and a peaceful life. I used the list to generate images for my scroll, some from photos, some small painting, others from the collage box, and then I added words and quotes as they came to me.

Once I got started, I couldn't stop thinking of images for the scroll. I loved my work as an art therapist and considered how lucky I was to be able to apply my love of art in the service of those in pain or need. And then there were so many friends, close by and far away, but present in my life on a daily basis. There were my best friends, the confidantes who helped me through life's challenges, helped me through loss or grieving, and shared shopping trips or a glass of wine. There were also colleagues who supported my work and challenged me to do better, and even telephone and Internet friends—editors, colleagues, and acquaintances—whom I rarely saw in person but with whom I felt a special bond.

The scroll set off a kind of chain reaction, and I began to give thanks for everything. I thought of the great crop of basil in the summer vegetable garden, the robin's nest in the apricot tree, and hearing an old favorite song on the radio. I was thankful for little things I had done in the past like sending a friend a box of wildflower seeds and hearing how year after year they reseeded and bloomed more beautifully than the year before. Or receiving a letter from a woman whom I had encouraged to write a book and getting word that it was about to be published.

The images and contents of the scroll grew and grew. I had to invent a way to add to the scroll; the original size I envisioned for my gratitude was now too small. So I began to glue on more paper as my gratitude scroll became an ongoing practice that I turn to when I want to express thanks for the abundance in my daily life.

A gratitude scroll and its images may set into motion an ancient soul wisdom for you: the more you are grateful for, the more will be given to you. Display it in your studio space or keep it rolled up on your desk where you can see it on a daily basis. During a time of emotional pain or suffering, looking beyond for gratitude can open your heart to the balance and wholeness it desperately needs. Using your creative source to imagine and express gratitude leads naturally to the experience of your true generosity. The more we make gratitude part of our day-to-day experiences, the more likely we are led to be generous to ourselves and others.

If you enjoy working in a book rather than on a scroll, use an image journal as your place of gratitude. Or try creating your own book with pages folded accordion style. Fold a number of pieces of heavy paper or card stock so that they look like blank greeting cards (or purchase blank cards at a stationery store). Carefully glue the back of one card to the front of another. Repeat this with as many cards as you like, making your accordion book as long as you wish. Glue cardboard or colored paper to the card surface on each end to form covers, and attach strings or ribbons to create a way to close your book. When you open the "accordion," all the pages can be displayed at once.

Make your gratitude scroll or book a long-term practice and add images and words that express your thankfulness on a regular basis. Think of it as a container for blessings that will awaken your heart to new things, increase your sense of abundance, and lead you to know the expansiveness of your generosity. Making visible your gratitude will help you to affirm what is good in life, bringing to consciousness what nourishes and supports you. You may find that it sets into motion a process of transformation that minimizes stress or loss while at the same time recovers a sense of emotional well-being and wholeness.

Mandalas: Making Order Out of Disorder

Our emotions sometimes throw us into chaos and nothing makes sense. At these times we often need to find a center amid the confusion, a way to pull together the scattered parts of life and find order.

The mandala is one such centering space for the self and the soul. *Mandala* is a Sanskrit word for "magic circle." For thousands of years the creation of circular, often geometric designs has been a part of spiritual practices around the world. Almost every culture has revered the power of the circle, and circular forms are found at sacred sites such as the prehistoric Stonehenge monument in Wiltshire, England, and the thirteenth-century circular labyrinth at the base of Chartres Cathedral in France. Spiritual seekers created mandalas to bring forth the sacred through images and have evoked the circle in ritual and art making for the purpose of transcendence, mindfulness, and wellness.

Making a mandala simply means creating an image within any circular space. Self-created mandalas are reflections of your inner self and are symbolic of your potential for change and transformation. When a mandala image suddenly turns up in your dreams or spontaneous art making, it is usually an indication of movement toward new self-knowledge.

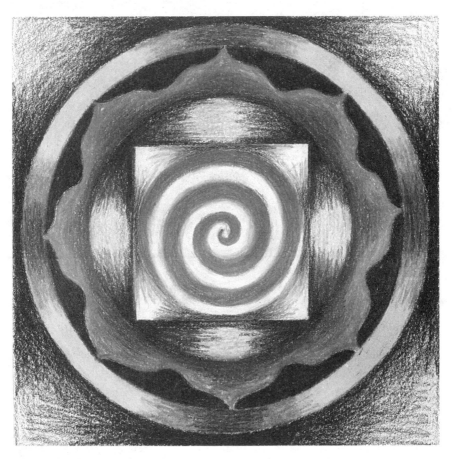

Mandala drawing by the author.

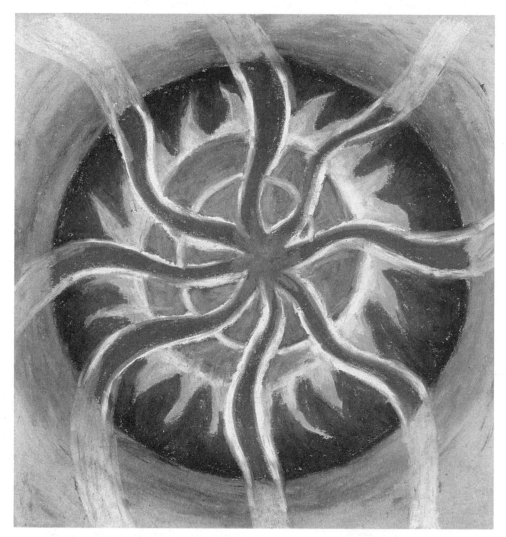

Mandala drawing by the author.

Jung is credited with introducing the Eastern concept of the mandala to Western thought and believed that this symbolic form represented the total personality, or Self. Art therapist Joan Kellogg spent
much of her life developing a system of understanding the wisdom
of the mandala, which she called the Great Round. She believes that
an intimate self-knowledge is intuitively reflected in the forms and

patterns, particularly about the current physical, emotional, and spiritual condition of the mandala maker.

In periods of intense stress or grieving, I have returned to the circle as a source of both wisdom and containment. Many years ago I was spontaneously attracted to working within the structure of a circle in my art at a time of emotional upheaval. I found myself wanting the control of a set of colored pencils and a circular space within the page of a small square drawing journal rather than my usual chalks or paints. For several months each day I worked at creating geometric designs in a circular format in that journal. Somehow it seemed right for me to use a ruler or a compass to carefully plan these images. Once in a while something more organic would emerge, like a spiral or snakelike shape or a maze of forms. Not only did coloring intricate patterns keep my mind focused, thus relieving my agitation, but I found that day by day my inner self became more peaceful even amid confusion or intense activity.

Mandala making, whether through drawing, painting, or three-dimensional media, can be similar to meditation. I find it easy to "slip off" both time and space when drawing a mandala. In my therapeutic work with individuals, I often suggest mandala drawing as a form of stress reduction for a troubled heart in times of emotional chaos.

If you are under emotional stress, I believe the best way to start mandala work is through drawing. The following materials are helpful in beginning your visual exploration:

- several sheets of 12-x-12-inch white paper (or a sketchbook of any size, but this is a good size to start with)
- oil pastels or colored chalks (try both; you may prefer one over the other, depending on how detailed you want to make your drawing)
- a round plate about 10 inches in diameter, for tracing a circle (or use a compass)
- a graphite pencil to sketch in any preliminary designs or images
- a ruler (for making precise straight lines)

Beginning on a sheet of white paper, use a pencil to trace the plate, or make a circle with a compass. You can also draw the circle freehand if you wish. With the drawing materials you have selected, fill in the circle in any way you want, using colors, lines, and forms. You can start at the center or the edges of the circle; you may also want to divide up the space within the circle in some way and position images or place colors within sections. You may either create a pattern or fill the space with random shapes and colors. If you want to extend your images outside the circle's boundary, feel free to do so. There is no right or wrong way to draw your mandala, so add to your drawing until you feel that it is complete.

When you have finished your drawing, mark the top of your paper or put an arrow on the back to indicate the orientation. Give your image a title if one comes to mind, writing it on the front or back of the drawing. You may also want to write a short description of the colors, shapes, patterns, or themes you see in your drawing.

Mandala drawings are particularly suited to drawing from the heart. Think of the inside of the circle as sacred space, and draw consciously from your heart, from a quiet place inside you that contains your true goodness and compassionate self. Try using the loving-kindness meditation described on page 161 as a prelude to mandala drawing. If no image comes to you, start by drawing an image of a simple heart shape within your circle, and let the rest grow from your intuition. Consider making this image your source for *metta* meditation or as the beginning of a series exploring your heart's capacity to give and receive loving-kindness.

Mandala Journals

A mandala journal is a special form of image journaling and is a practice that is both soothing and stress reducing. Staying with drawing or painting within a circle is containing, structured, and satisfying and can be particularly healing during times of crisis or loss. Keeping such a journal is a transformative practice because your mandala images will change and evolve over time. There may be days or weeks when you find your images or symbols stay pretty much the same; or you may feel that you cannot go forward or away from certain images that you have created. But if you stay with the practice on a regular basis, you will begin to see, as with other forms of spontaneous imagery, surprising changes in the color, pattern, and content of your drawings.

The following suggestions may help you get started in creating a mandala journal:

1. Select a square format, which will best contain circular images. Buy a square sketchbook, available in a variety of sizes at art or stationery stores, or have a copy shop cut paper to the size you specify and put a spiral binding on it for you.

2. Consider what type of art materials you will be using before you select or create your journal. For example, if you want to use colored pencils, a smaller sketchbook (6 x 6 or 8 x 8 inches) would be a good size. If you are using oil pastels or chalk pastels, a larger sketchbook (8 x 8 inches or more) is appropriate. For a serious practice of mandala drawing, treat yourself to a very nice set of professional colored pencils or oil pastels in at least 24 colors; if you shop at an art supply store, you can also buy extra colors in open stock.

3. Because creating a mandala is a quiet, meditative experience, try playing your favorite relaxing or dreamy music to inspire your imagination and open your creative source. Some suggestions for music are listed in the resources section at the end of this book.

4. If you are having a hard time getting started on a particular day, try dividing your circle into parts: a quadrant, a square within the circumference, or a series of free-form shapes. Go outside the space if you wish.

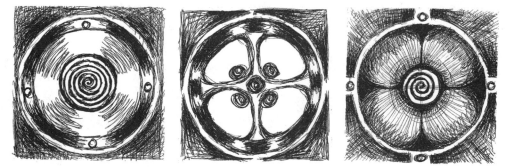

Entry from a mandala journal.

Don't worry if your mandala designs are not symmetrical or carefully balanced; go ahead and experiment with free-form or organic designs within the circle. Think of your mandala drawings as your self emerging: in life, we are rarely completely orderly, balanced, and perfect. What is in our hearts flows to its own special rhythm, sometimes discordant and at other times a finely tuned melody. Let your mandala journal become a reflection for the emotions that are within and flowing through you right now, and enjoy the process.

RENEWING AND RESTORING THE HEART

Here are several additional transformational practices that can deepen your capacity to use art expression for emotional healing and balance.

Take regular art breaks for emotional health and wellness. Andrew Weil, M.D., an expert on wellness practices, notes that something as simple as a weekly bouquet of flowers or a work of art displayed within one's environment can enhance a positive sense of self. Use these types of images to take a mental break from your distress and create a sanctuary within your home that includes a little bit of natural imagery and aesthetics. In addition, make it a habit to visit a place of beauty or an art gallery on a regular basis as care for the heart.

Maintain your feelings journal. Sustaining the practice of image journaling helps you to continue your process of sensory awareness and encourages emotions to come to the surface, flowing through you rather than becoming toxic to your well-being. Try this practice as a daily activity, or simply keep an ongoing feelings journal that you can go to when you need to express, understand, or receive wisdom from your creative source.

Use trauma or loss as a mobilizing force for artistic and creative growth. Although there are many times in my life I would have preferred to escape emotional pain and suffering, these times have also been catalysts for creativity. In the weeks following the death of my mother, I found myself wanting the comfort of my studio and the escape that paints and paper provided. While initially my creative source was a refuge from the pain and grief, it also opened me to new ways of expression and imagination that I would not have experienced if I had not taken the risk to trust the process. A time of loss became a catalyst for new creative directions and deepened my connection to my soul's palette.

GOING FURTHER

The poet Rainer Maria Rilke said, "You must give birth to your images, they are the future waiting to be born."[3] I believe that making images also makes tangible the past and present, and, by doing so, we are freed to create a future when trauma or loss is holding us back. Our creative source can be both a conduit to and a catalyst for emotional well-being, wholeness, and healing.

Art and imagination are medicines for emotional distress. However, while artistic creativity can be a companion on the journey, when undergoing stress or trauma, don't go it alone. It may be important to have a witness for your art expressions and experiences. This may be a professional therapist, a family physician, a pastoral counselor, or a support group that understands your trauma or loss.

In the next chapter, you will learn how to continue renewing and restoring your heart through using your creative source to nurture your spirit.

NINE

Nurturing the Sacred

*I*n this era of high-priced galleries and competitive celebrity artists, we sometimes forget that art's primary role since the dawn of humanity has been to nourish the sacred dimension of life. From Tibetan mandalas to Japanese gardening and architecture to Navaho sandpainting ceremonies, art is still a form of soul awakening for traditional cultures. By involving yourself in art and imagination, even in simple ways, you attend to both spirit and soul and come to know yourself more fully and deeply.

Visualize a familiar artwork such as Michelangelo's *Pietà* statue or Van Gogh's brilliant painting *Starry Night* and you experience how images engage your spiritual nature. Simply by witnessing these images you intuitively know that they embody spirit. By tapping your own creative source, you can also encounter that same inspirational force in your own life. We are all yearning to put into tangible form what it is to be spirit and to witness its miracles. Artistic expression, even through the humblest materials, is a way of experiencing and knowing spirit.

Thomas Moore, author of *Care of the Soul*, stresses the spiritual benefits of art as a source of contemplation. Art making and the creative source are ways to touch spirit, call it forth, and encounter the sacred. And the Indian spiritual master Meher Baba has stated the connection between art and spirituality this way: "Art, when inspired with love, leads to higher realms, and that art will open for you the inner life. When you paint, you forget everything except your object. When you are engrossed in it, you are lost in it; when you are lost in it, your ego diminishes; and when the ego diminishes, Love Infinite appears; and when love is created, God is attained. So you see how art can lead one to find Infinite God."[1]

One of the central purposes of artistic creativity, then, is spiritual practice, a way of awakening to our true nature and the meaning of life. In this chapter you will learn how you can nurture the sacred within through artistic expression, how to initiate a deeper connection to spiritual wisdom, and why art making is a path to compassion and peace.

THE SACREDNESS OF THE CREATIVE SOURCE

I believe that spirit is the inner experience of the sacred in our lives. We all have encountered the sacred at some time, and when we have, images are almost always involved. Consider a magnificent sunset when the sky is ablaze with color, the birth of a child, a sudden spring rain, the wonder of the ocean waves, or the peacefulness of a temple or church. Our visual memories can also call forth that which is spiritual. We may have a mental image of someone who helped us during a time of desperation, loss, or tragedy, or how we felt safe as a child in the lap of a grandparent.

Hildegard of Bingen, a twelfth-century German abbess, is a wonderful example of art as a conduit of spirit. While enveloped in mystical visions, Hildegard was moved to create icons from her visions. When she was forty-two years old, a fiery light of tremendous brightness coming from heaven poured into her mind and heart. So strong were these experiences that she had to retreat to her bed. From that point on she felt the need to enkindle other hearts so that imagination, creativity, forgiveness, and contrition would flow throughout the world. Hildegard describes her experiences as a spiritual awakening that stirred the divine spark within her and led her to create art and music as a result.

The well-known neurologist and author Oliver Sacks believes that Hildegard's visions were associated with intense migraine headaches, the classic symptoms of which include visual "auras" or images of light and debilitating illness requiring bed rest. But no matter what the medical implications, Hildegard's visions led her to seek out the mysteries of creativity and imagination and to inspire others with her artistry during her century and in contemporary times. She turned what could have been merely an incapacitating illness into creative images of God and spirit that have touched the souls of people for centuries.

Another creative genius who has enhanced our understanding of spirit is William Blake, the mystic artist and poet of the eighteenth–nineteenth century, who was said to have conversed with angels and received painting instructions from entities beyond the earthly plane of existence. He said his work came from Divine Imagination. Contemporary artists have found their own paths to spirituality through art and image. Wassily Kandinsky sought to cultivate the sacred in his paintings, the later works of Mark Rothko touch on spiritual journeys and realizations, and the spirit of nature is the essence of Andy Goldsworthy's environmental works.

Creativity has continually been defined by artists as a spiritual practice and even a form of prayer. It doesn't matter whether you believe that art making is divinely inspired or is simply an expression of your inner awareness; both are ultimately enlightening. What is important is that in creating images we call forth spirit, and in knowing spirit, we bring well-being to our souls.

ART AS TRANSCENDENCE

When art making becomes a true wellness practice, it is often related to the experience of transcendence. Transcendence is often viewed as a condition of rising above and away from worldly life, into some lofty spiritual realm. But I believe that transcendence means finding a place within oneself where spirit resides and then carrying that spiritual self back into life, no matter what obstacles exist. It is the place where the heart is most open and where your creative source flows freely, honestly, and with confidence. It is being in oneness with your creativity, art making, and imagination.

I have been humbled to witness art's transcendent function by watching adults and children make images. Among these individuals, one in particular stands out. For a year I had the privilege of working with Joanne, a woman who survived breast cancer for four years, only to have the cancer return later to other parts of her body. After a series of tests and examinations, her prognosis was not favorable. The disease had spread to her spine, pelvis, and liver, and effective treatment options had been exhausted.

Joanne came to measure her life in months rather than the years that most of us expect from life, and she began to paint with an urgency of one who knows there is not much time left. When she could not come to the local cancer wellness house to work with me, I went to her home and to her bedside if necessary. Despite an intravenous injection that dulled her with painkillers on bad days, she never stopped to feel sorry for herself and continued to create bold paintings with large washes of color. Her experience of life-threatening illness gave her wisdom about life beyond her thirty-two years and a deeply personal understanding of how art making enhances life, even in the face of death.

A special relationship evolved between us over the course of our work together. I offered a therapist's support and reflection and provided encouragement and advice from one artist to another. We usually shared a cup of ginger tea as our ritual at the end of the session, along with conversation about local art events and people we both knew. Each and every meeting with Joanne taught me a valuable lesson. Even confronted with death and disabled by pain, or medical treatment, she was still motivated to express herself and, in that process, transcend her illness and heal her spirit even without hope of a cure or remission.

Sharing the experience of art making with Joanne also offered me a form of transcendence through becoming one with her in the creative source. Often, I shared moments of being deeply connected to her and I was filled with compassion and gratitude for the times I spent in her company witnessing her artistic process enfold. Her courage to be in the moment despite the constant threat of physical death allowed me to see Joanne as spirit rather than as simply a person with cancer. I think this is an experience of the Divine being manifested, and it is a gift we can give ourselves through art making, both as creators and as witnesses to the creative process.

The most important lesson for me, one I relearn again and again, is that creativity and healing are gateways to spirit and to wellness. Finding your authentic voice through art takes you to this portal, and putting your trust into the process guides you to a place within you that touches spirit and restores soul.

RECOGNIZING THE VOICE OF YOUR SPIRIT

There are some specific ways I have found to draw closer to spirit in my own life. Some of them have soothed my spirit, while others have cultivated compassion and loving-kindness toward myself and others. At other times, art images have become prayers, spiritual intentions made on behalf of specific people, groups, or communities.

Spirit Guides and Guardians

As a child, I grew up learning about guardian angels who watched over me on my way home from school, on the playground, or when I had the measles. I have a crisp memory of a holographic print of a guardian angel hovering over two children as they crossed a treacherous bridge that was on my bedroom wall as a very young child. My godmother, who gave me the print, told me numerous stories of how these invisible beings kept us from harm and how each of us had at least one whose personal assignment was to watch over our daily lives. A large part of my feelings of security as a child in a poor family came from believing that I was always cared for, beyond the boundaries of what I could see but vividly present in my imagination. The image of a guarding angelic being was one of my first contacts with something divine, both within and outside myself.

As an adult I have felt a guardian's actual presence. When I have experienced emotionally difficult times, I have encountered my Italian grandmother and a deceased cousin who was my playmate in childhood. Sometimes I felt the need to have a conversation with these guardians, and at other times their presence was enough to sustain me. In one moment of deep despair, my Italian grandmother, whom I had never met, cradled me in her arms one night as I was falling asleep. It was the peace that I desperately needed at that time, and her presence was one of the few experiences that could give me the rest I needed. My cousin I imagine as my true guardian angel, who has been present whenever I have experienced the dark night of the soul.

Whether you label these encounters as inner voices, visions, or a visitation from the dearly departed, what is important is how these sensory experiences touch and nurture spirit in times of distress, pain, or suffering. For me, these are images that connect me to what is sacred and are present to help me experience my own spirit in new and life-giving ways. They help me to rise beyond pain and suffering and cultivate an authentic relationship to the divine within myself and others.

Sometimes, I have created my own guardians to help me through a rough spot or two. During the months after I decided to leave a faculty post, I went through a time when I felt alone and unsure of my decision to leave academia for work as a therapist. I wanted something to guide me and support me during this transition to a career that was yet to be defined. I spent several weeks constructing a series of small guardian figures from scraps of balsa wood and found objects. I based them on the idea of spirit dolls, American Indian sculptures representing guardians who inhabit the forests, mountains, and rivers. Often made of recycled materials, the dolls may be adorned with healing herbs such as sweet grass, sage, or lavender. Their intention is to bring power and peace, to guard and protect, but they also embody our own intuition and wisdom and help us to follow our dreams, especially those that require a difficult journey.

Try making an image of your guardian, one you have already encountered or one you imagine. Create it in the tradition of the spirit doll, using recycled fabric, scrap paper, or natural objects such as feathers, twigs, seedpods, or small shells. Start with an armature, the framework for the doll; this can be a piece of wood, a tree branch, a coat hanger wire, a wooden dowel, or an old-fashioned wooden clothespin. Be spontaneous and free in how you fashion and embellish your guardian. You may want to build a simple platform or box for it out of cardboard or wood to give it a special home and enshrine it.

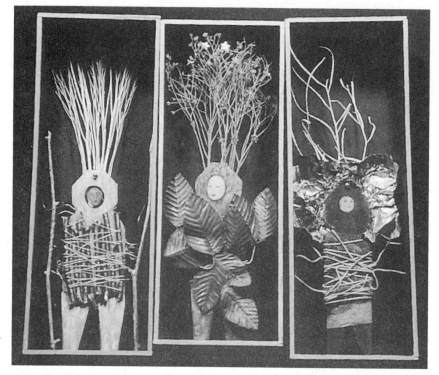

Guardian figures.

Place your figure where you can see it every day. You may want to place it beside your bed, in the tradition of Guatemalan worry dolls, or in a prominent spot in your studio space. A friend of mine put her guardian figure at the top of her front doorway to bless and protect all that enter her home. Think of your figure as an intention to bring good feelings, support, and spiritual wholeness into your life and the lives of family members and friends.

GETTING TO YOUR SPIRITUAL CENTER

One consistent symbol that we humans have returned to repeatedly on our spiritual quests is the circle, for the purpose of finding within us the center, core, and heart of that which is sacred. The following activities and practices will help you to get to your spiritual center by using the image of a circle as your starting point.

Mandalas as a Spiritual Practice

Mandala drawing, described in the previous chapter, not only helps make order out of emotional chaos, it is also a spiritual practice. As a form of sacred art, it has been used both for finding one's spiritual center and for reflection on the nature of existence. Tibetan monks spend days creating intricate mandalas from colored sand, recapturing a ritual handed down over generations.

Joan Kellogg believes that a black background guides you to naturally tap the spiritual dimension. It also encourages you to use lighter colors, such as white, yellow, and pastels, than on white paper; these colors often appear as luminous on a dark or black ground. Try the following activities to explore the potential of mandalas to take you to your spiritual center.

◆ Use colored pencils or oil pastels on black paper. You may have to go to an art store to find black drawing paper or board suitable for drawing. Alternatively, black gesso on paper or canvas is good if you would rather work with paints. (See page 169 for size suggestions.)

◆ With a black surface as a background, try using white pencils or oil pastels only, or use pencils or markers in white and metallic colors (gold, bronze, and silver). Using these colors on black evokes the idea of an image emerging from the darkness, just as the universe emerged from the darkness of space.

◆ Make mandala images inspired by spiritual traditions, such as images of gods and goddess, nature, or religious symbols that are significant to you. Again, use a black surface and light or shiny colors. If no specific images come to mind, simply work with the colors and let figures and forms emerge organically.

Taking the Spiral Path

A spiritual path is often depicted in art and lore through the image of a spiral. The motion of a spiral circles around, seeming to move

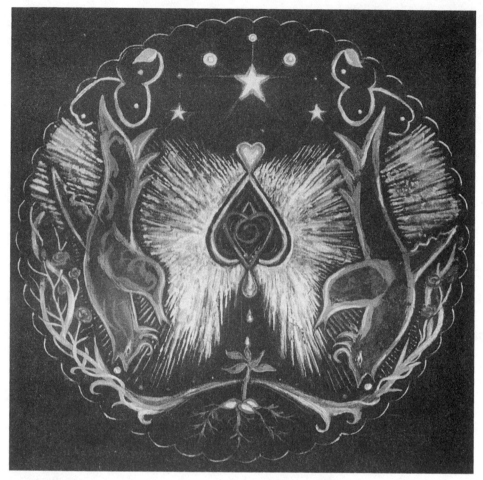

A mandala drawing on black background by Michael Campanelli.

backward yet rising to a higher level. Spiritual development appears to take a similar course, as we often find ourselves circling back to experiences or feelings we thought we had finished with, yet now we re-experience them with (we hope) a greater understanding. The spiral is an image that suggests circular movement toward and away from its center and is present in a range of phenomena, from the movements of galaxies to the act of stirring a pot of soup on the stove.

The circular or spiral movement known as circumambulation has significance in both religion and psychology. Ritual circumambulation is practiced in many traditions: the Japanese wind around Mount Fuji, for example, and Muslims on pilgrimage to Mecca circle the holy Kaaba. Following a spiral path is like the passing of the years of our lives; our worldview gets a little bit wider and the spiral expands outward with each cycle. Jung believed that the psychological process of circumambulation was an aid in actualizing the Self. In Jungian psychology, to circumambulate means to circle around an image or experience and interpret it from many different points of view.

Because of its universality as a symbol, the spiral has much to teach us. I go to it frequently in my own image work, especially when I feel stuck or confused. It has a transformative quality to it and is said to embody the desire to move toward wholeness and to contact the divine imagination and one's creative energies. For this reason, it is an image that people often enjoy experimenting with in art making.

In recent years, the spiral as a path to spiritual awakening and wellness has resonated within our contemporary culture in the form of the labyrinth, an ancient pattern used for meditation, whether as an actual path that one walks in a garden or retreat center or even a virtual labyrinth on the Internet. The image of the labyrinth, a variation of the spiral, is being re-created in backyards, hospital gardens, playgrounds, and places of worship. More than a million people have explored Grace Cathedral's indoor labyrinth in San Francisco since its installation in 1991, and millions of others have visited labyrinths throughout the world in recent years.

Most labyrinth enthusiasts say they have come to find something profound in the path and in the center of the circle. They experience a meditation in motion, combining mindful walking with the experience of spiritual centering and a sense of well-being. When you concentrate on the spiral path, your pace naturally slows, your breathing deepens, and your mind becomes calm. There is a kind of circular logic to the labyrinth; unlike a maze, which has dead ends and false leads, it has only a single path, which one follows to the center and back. It is a metaphor for a healing journey or a symbolic pilgrimage.

There are a variety of activities and practices that can help you to experience the transformative potential of the labyrinth:

Walk the labyrinth. At a local cancer wellness community in my city, a labyrinth has been created in the adjoining carport so that people can walk it year-round. Chances are there is a labyrinth near you, too;

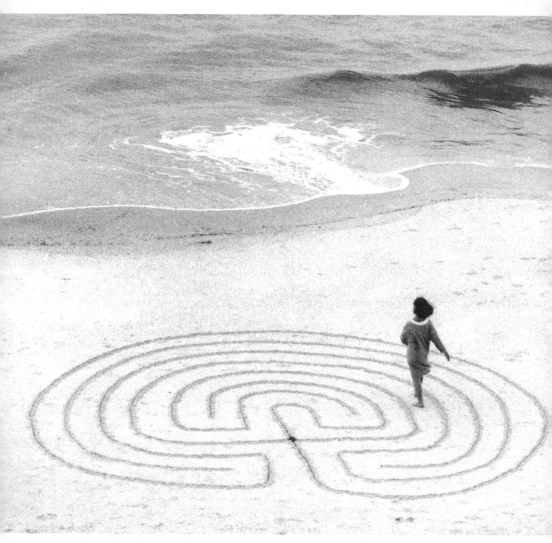

"Seaside Labyrinth" by Annette Reynolds.

if not, there are numerous sources, both in books and on Internet sites, that give excellent instructions on how to create and use a life-size labyrinth. Many labyrinths are created in backyards with whatever is available—stones, sand, concrete stepping stones, or wood. Check local art centers, churches, or wellness programs to see if a labyrinth has been created for the purpose of walking.

Try a virtual labyrinth. Visit one of the many Internet sites that have virtual labyrinths. (See resources section at end of book.) You can often print out one of these small labyrinths right from your computer and experience a "finger walk" through its spiral path. Tracing a labyrinth path with your index finger (the nondominant hand is recommended) can facilitate quiet centering and create a sense of inner peace.

Make a mini-labyrinth. Try making your own spiral path or miniature labyrinth. Get a square piece of cardboard, foam core, or fiberboard (found in home improvement stores) at least 20 x 20 inches; this will serve as the background for your labyrinth. You will also need at least a 20-foot length of thin cotton clothesline, white glue or a glue gun, and materials to embellish your labyrinth such as paints, small stones or shells, collage materials, and glitter.

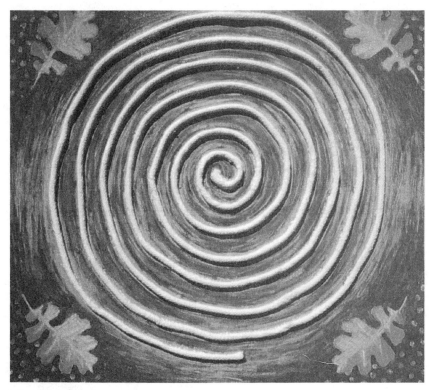

Mini-labyrinth for meditation.

With a pencil, start at the center of your background and draw a freehand spiral, working your way outward. This pencil line will be your guideline for gluing the clothesline and will create a dimensional spiral. While a spiral is not exactly the same as the spiral maze of a true labyrinth, your image will approximate the qualities of an actual labyrinth. Add other materials to your spiral design if you wish, or paint the outer borders with your own special images or favorite colors.

When the work is complete, try a "finger walk" as described above, using the index finger of your nondominant hand. I find that several slow repetitions of a finger walk through my minilabyrinth can calm me down after a busy day and provide an experience similar to walking a full-size labyrinth. Use your minilabyrinth in this way as a daily transformational practice or simply spend time meditating on the spiral image, offering loving-kindness to your spiritual self.

Calling Forth Windhorse

Ritual and intention are important aspects of caring for and healing spirit. Tibetan Buddhists have a sacred tradition that is based on the element of wind sending their prayers into the atmosphere to reach the ears of supernatural beings. To assist the process, they create prayer flags, colorful cloths with symbols of enlightenment and prayers or mantras that the wind distributes to the world each time it comes in contact with the flag. The Tibetan word for prayer flag is *lung-ta*, which translates literally as "windhorse," which symbolizes the uplifting energy of spirit.

Traditionally, prayer flags are used to promote peace, compassion, strength, and wisdom. They are also said to bring happiness and good health to all who hang the flags as well as to their families, loved ones, neighbors, nearby strangers, and enemies. The prayers of a flag become a permanent part of the universe as the images fade from wind and sun. Just as life moves on and is replaced by new life, Tibetans renew their hopes for the world by continually mounting new flags alongside of the old. This act symbolizes a welcoming of life's changes and an acknowledgment that all beings are part of a greater, ongoing circle of life.

The Tibetan master Khenpo Rinpoche says we can raise wind energy both mentally and physically, but it is more important through intention and prayer than anything else.[2] Mentally, we raise windhorse through developing compassion, loving-kindness, and wisdom. When you have confidence and fearlessness in your mind, that is mental windhorse.

Create a prayer flag. With respect for the spiritual tradition of the prayer flag, consider ways you can make a similar image that will carry your spirit's intention in the form of a flag or other media. Traditional prayer flags are blue, white, green, red, or gold cotton cloth decorated with religious symbols and framed with the words of a prayer. You can use markers on fabric to create an image of your own spirit's intention and write your prayer around the border of the piece. Intentions such as "Let there be world peace" or "Please protect all lost souls" are often written on flags, but any intention of a spiritual or compassionate nature is appropriate. Attach your flag to your porch railing or use a pole or tree branch to hang it.

Call forth your own windhorse. Consider other ways of creating images using the prayer flag as a metaphor. I participated in a powerful ritual at a funeral for a young child who had died from bone cancer. At an outdoor ceremony we were each given a colorful balloon to color with felt pens and to write a prayer for the child on a small piece of cloth that was attached to the balloon string. Together, in an open field, we released the balloons and watched them ascend to the sky. As the wind blew, our prayers were released to the heavens. The loving-prayer balloons were like a variation of the prayer flag, a joyful, creative gesture that uplifted the spirits of the mourners.

On another occasion, a group of people with similar intentions for a common goal to raise a specific amount of money for a charity decided to write their prayers for donations on paper. The intentions were put in a metal container, which was then placed in a small bonfire. The container had a small slit in it, and as the papers burned, the prayers symbolically rose as smoke toward heaven. While the ritual quality of the event was spiritually inspiring, the secondary miracle of the ceremony was in receiving twice the amount of monetary donations expected.

COMMIT RANDOM ACTS OF ART

In Buddhism, a powerful expression of compassion in action is given by a *bodhisattva*, a person who has dedicated his or her life to the service of others and vowed to ease the suffering of others whenever possible. The Dalai Lama points out that taking the bodhisattva vow doesn't force one into a life of service to others, but it does set a life path for offering aid and acts of charity. This can be donating money, delivering food to an elderly person, or volunteering on a hospital ward. However, a bodhisattva vow can also involve "random acts of kindness," simple actions on behalf of others, often performed anonymously.

Since childhood I have been engaged in what I now call "random acts of art." My mother started me on this path by encouraging me to make artistic creations for others. One winter I made potted plants by cutting empty dish detergent containers in half to form a simple pot, painted them with acrylic paints, and placed soil and a narcissus bulb inside each. I carefully watched for signs of the bulbs' germination in our hall closet. When the first green shoots appeared, my mother and I went to a nursing home to give several of the residents a plant in one of my decorated containers.

When I was in junior high school, my history teacher had a heart attack and was hospitalized for several weeks. My classmates collected money to buy him a present, but somehow I didn't feel satisfied with just buying him a wool scarf. Instead, I spent one evening making a collage of historic figures from early American history, each captioned with something humorous and extending wishes for a speedy recovery. Because it was too large to be sent by mail, my father and I brought it to the intensive care unit at the hospital. The teacher's wife called me the next day to gratefully thank me for helping to bring her husband out of his postoperative depression by bringing the collage, which not only moved him and made him laugh but also revived his spirit by touching on the subjects that interested and excited him.

Creative gifts like these are ways to share spirit with others, at the same time lifting our own. I myself have been the delighted recipient of many random acts of art from others over the years. A dear friend who makes beautiful decorated gourds embellished with African designs surprised me with one of her creations in the mail. Another friend sent a thank-you in the form of a hand-drawn card with a favorite scone recipe on the back. Her rough but colorful sketch showed the scones as they appear when served in her home on Sunday mornings. A long-time friend and colleague in California occasionally sends a Post-it note with a quick cartoon of herself on it; I have saved these caricatures for ten years now and look forward with anticipation to receiving more of these random acts of art in the future.

The standard operating procedure of guardian angels is a wonderful model for random acts of art. Guardian angels are beings who appear on the scene, give assistance, and then disappear as mysteriously as they arrived. The anonymity of angels has inspired my own random acts of art on behalf of others over the years. Once a month for a year, I sent hand-painted and collaged postcards anonymously to an old college friend who lived out of state. We were rarely able to see each other over the years but kept in touch by phone or exchanging holiday letters. At the time of his retirement from teaching, I wanted

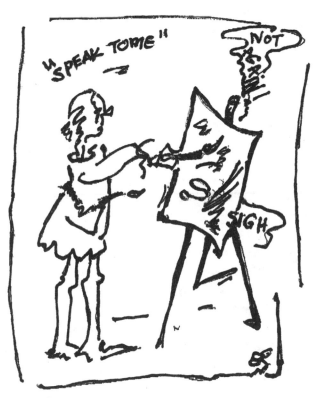

Speak to Me! Not Again! Caricature by Shirley Riley.

to celebrate his accomplishments and thank him for his friendship and help during graduate school. Those simple handmade postcards carried my good intentions for his life transition, and he was baffled but pleased (I learned later) to keep finding the mysterious paintings and collages in his mailbox. It took him a long time to figure out who the anonymous postcard artist was because I sent them from different cities or had friends post them on their travels. To this day we still surprise each other with little pieces of art, mailed anonymously to keep up the guardian-angel tradition.

I think random acts of art are good examples of the true purpose of art making—making day-to-day life special through creativity. In making art for others I am also doing a service to myself. It makes me feel good, it stimulates my own creative process, and it nourishes my soul in wonderful and gratifying ways.

A random act of art can be as simple as doodle or a photo, or can be a more thoughtful work given without strings or expectations. Take time to frame an image to give to a friend or decorate a set of cloth dinner napkins with fabric paints for the next person who invites you to a meal at her home—it doesn't matter what it is, because the old saying is true—it really is the thought that counts. Perhaps you know someone in your life who is suffering, sad, or ill who you feel could benefit from the gift of an image or handmade object from you. The surprise gift of a genuine act of art is a potent symbol that is particularly meaningful to someone who is going through stress or loss.

Try sending a visual act of kindness to someone who is not a friend, who might even be an opponent or even someone you hate. The bodhisattva vow includes having loving-kindness and compassion for those we consider enemies. A couple of years ago I was confronted with my own dislike for a colleague who I felt treated me unjustly and without regard for my feelings. I wallowed around in sensations of frustration, anger, and desire for downright revenge for quite a few months. I tried to practice loving-kindness meditation, actively sending good wishes and compassion to this woman. Mostly, it was not successful and actually stimulated even more unpleasant feelings.

I realized that I had to free myself from these feelings or they would consume me. I decided to send her two images in compassion and kindness. The first was a sketch of my flower garden in summer and in full-bloom of daisies, Russian sage, liatris, and marigolds. The second was a container of wildflower seeds for her to plant as a metaphor for new beginnings and an end to the discord between us.

I never heard a word from her about these gestures. But I found that her lack of response didn't matter. I had been liberated through my own "acts of art." Taking the time to create an image of healing and growth for her came back to me and gave me the grace to find forgiveness and understanding, let go, and move forward.

Try using the practice of loving-kindness and art making along with the intention to create a piece of art for another person. Gradually expand the focus of your intention for art making to include others. Start with someone in your life who has truly cared for you. Visualize that person, extend your *metta* meditation to include him or her, and use this feeling as an inspiration for your creative source. Eventually, and with practice, you can gradually begin to include others—friends, neighbors, and community members. Try adding in and experimenting with the most difficult people in your life, wishing that they, too, be filled with loving-kindness and peace, trying to hold this feeling within your art making. As you silently practice this way of making art through a place of compassion for yourself and for others, you will begin to feel a wonderful connection with them that will lift your spirit, calm your soul, and connect you to the true loving nature of your heart.

Taking a bodhisattva vow to art does not mean overlooking yourself in service of others. You will not feel satisfied if you only make images to give away all the time. There is a pleasure and joy in making images for yourself, too. Remember that nourishing your own creative source makes it possible to unconditionally share the soul's palette with others.

Creating Images of Compassion

One way that we get in touch with compassion within ourselves is through empathizing with the suffering of others. In my office I keep a photograph that conveys a powerful sense of both suffering and service within the image. It is a photo of my Italian relatives, my uncle Nicola Malchiodi, and his son, my cousin Luigi. Nicola is in his bed in our family homestead in Grondone, high in the mountains south of Piacenza. My uncle is very old and has been so ill for the last few years that he cannot walk up and down stairs any longer, and Luigi now carries him upstairs to his bed each night and downstairs to the kitchen hearth. When Luigi told me this, I asked him, "How can you do this night after night? You work hard each day, for long hours doing physical labor. Then you come home and care for your father. You must be exhausted every day." Luigi's answer was very simple and sincere. He replied that when he was a very young child, his father carried him upstairs to his bedroom each night, and now he is returning his father's love for him by doing the same for him.

I often look at this photograph before I begin working with people in therapy or leading a workshop. It is a visual reminder to me of the compassion that exists through service to others and also is an image of suffering because my uncle is very old and infirm in the photo. It brings both sadness to my heart and compassion through remembering Luigi's selfless service to his father. Ultimately, I think it helps me to stay connected to those inner resources that help me to listen with respect to people's problems and to find the compassion within myself to witness others' suffering with humility.

Collect images that help you stay connected to your own sense of compassion and inspire you to serve others in your life. These can be photos of those who inspire service, such as Mother Teresa, a favorite patron saint such as Saint Francis, or a religious leader like Martin Luther King, Jr., or the Dalai Lama. You may find images of children or animals that evoke a sense of compassion and loving-kindness. Inspirational words or quotes are another good source. Try pulling both images and words together into a collage or simply arrange them in an informal composition that you can tack up on a wall and add to as you find other pictures.

TRANSFORMATIONAL PRACTICES TO NURTURE SPIRIT

In addition to the activities and practices already mentioned, try the following to deepen your experience of art making as care for your spirit:

Use images to soothe and restore the spirit. Continue to develop your studio space or some part of your home or office as a sacred place. Select and arrange images and objects that generate a sense of transcendence and prompt appreciation, gratitude, and compassion. A luminous mandala created on black paper; a few Zen-like brushstrokes; a simple altar with a deity, family photos, or objects of nature; or a collection of prayer beads or other objects that awaken your spiritual nature.

Connect with the images of nature. Nature offers a traditional path from image to spirit. Moses, Jesus, Muhammad, and the authors of the Hindu Vedas were all seekers of spirit in nature's solitude. Retreat to the forest is the trademark of holy individuals like Buddha and the divine incarnations Krishna and Rama. Saint Francis has been dubbed the patron saint of ecology because of his love of nature as a path to peace and spirit. Thoreau's writing is flooded with passages that reflect the serenity of the natural world.

The wisdom of nature and its connection to spirit is something that we all can engage through communing with and working with images of nature in the artistic process. Some of my most spirit-filled drawings and paintings have come as a result of encounters with the ocean, canyons, and the trees and deer in my own backyard. By running your hand over a granite boulder, collecting seedpods and twigs, or just poking through the woods for spring blooms, open yourself to what William Blake called "eternity in a grain of sand." Maintain a garden, dig out a new plot for perennials, take snapshots of flowers and vegetables, collect leaves and buds to use in a collage, or sit outdoors to make quick sketches of a landscape or vista. There is a spiritual wisdom in both the art of nature and the nature of art; making images of nature is a way to know spirit.

Simply enjoy the mystery. Spirit fills us with awe and wonder. We may be moved to a quiet, inner place of peace by it, feel lucky or blessed, or even glimpse another reality that we rarely see. We may be filled with a deep gratitude and appreciation for the Divine. But most of all, spirit evokes a sense of mystery, for it cannot be fathomed by the mind—it can only be experienced.

The creative source within resonates with a similar mystery. We enter the mystery each time we call on our creative source, whether we are facing a piece of paper with a pen or putting the first few brush-strokes on a canvas. We may not know what we want to create, but something always emerges from us as image, whether through art making, imagination, or dreams. What is important is to trust ourselves to take the risk of self-expression. In doing so, we immediately begin a journey of exploration that brings with it inevitable surprises. Along the way we may even find the answers to a problem or question that has baffled us for months, if we are willing to give ourselves over to the mystery of the creative process. Moments of astonishment or wonder are common to the arts. In order to enjoy these moments, be sure to leave a little room for the mystery to happen.

§

Sometimes the best way to nurture spirit is to simply let your creative source guide you like an invisible companion, whatever medium you choose. As Pat Allen, artist and art therapist, reminds us, "To create means to walk on holy ground, to engage with the Divine, and to experience it moving through me to manifestation. . . . This is not possible if I am trying to manage or direct this force, if I am trying to meet the needs of my ego by way of creative work."[3] Paradoxically, it is by learning to let go of ego, expectations, and outcome in the artistic process that the most powerful work on behalf of spirit occurs. When we are consciously trying to have an insight or heal, our egos are doing the work. If we can let the ego step aside, spirit takes care of the outcome. It is in that moment that we accept the mystery and allow much more important forces to intervene and healing to take place.

The power of art to nurture and heal spirit is most exquisitely demonstrated when we join with each other to make art together. The next chapter explains how creating together and extending your studio to neighborhoods, communities, and the world is a manifestation of the soul's palette that unites us in the mystery and the miracle of art making as a wellness practice.

TEN

Sharing the Artist Within

rt usually happens behind closed doors, where the artist is isolated from the "real world." The studio, whether a room or a drawing journal, can be an oasis from stress, an emotional refuge, a source of inner wisdom, or a place of spiritual renewal. The sacredness of working in solitude is a large part of the power of creativity to restore, repair, and replenish the soul.

While there is no doubt that your creative source can be nurtured in your own studio, I believe that artistic creativity is also meant to be communal and has the potential to heal groups of individuals. In both ancient and contemporary cultures, people gather in groups to experience and use art to heal and make whole not only one person but also the larger community. Visual rituals, images, and the use of imagination have always been called upon to care for the collective as well as the personal soul.

By sharing your creative spirit in a larger community, you extend your artistic wisdom to others in positive and transformative ways while healing yourself. Your artistic creativity is a gift to yourself, but by sharing it, it is also a gift to your community and the world.

The way to truly honor oneself is through community. In this way, the soul is nourished by communal values, traditions, rituals, and exchanges. Connectedness is what brings us to discover authenticity, content, and meaning. In this chapter you will identify how you can continue your journey with the creative process through creating art with others and how you can use your artistic creativity to be part of a community solution to serve others in need.

WE ARE ALL IN IT TOGETHER

There is no argument that we humans live on a planet whose growth and, ultimately, survival are dependent on interdependence with all living beings. Ignoring our interconnectness in the world has led to the potential for the destruction of the environment and the proliferation of war, violence, and abuse on individual and collective levels. Buddhism teaches a concept called "dependent origination," which means that everything that exists is dependent on the concurrent existence of everything else in the world. Each of us is part of this dynamic whole and, in a sense, part of the same organism. As in the movie *It's a Wonderful Life*, if any one person or part of the overall picture is removed, everything changes. Equally, if we make an action or intention, everything changes, too.

Despite this knowledge, we often find ourselves directed by society toward a notion of individualism and an individual consciousness and soul. Scholars and philosophers have repeatedly challenged the idea that soul exists only inside of us and that consciousness is truly a collective. Satish Kumar observes that in struggling so hard to heal the individual soul, the soul of the world (the *animus mundi*) undergoes great suffering, pain, and damage. He believes that we must reconnect with the soul of the world, and in doing so, we will naturally heal our own souls. Kumar says that when we use our artistic creativity, we are part of the great flow of all art making and become part of a larger continuum of healing. He believes that art's primary function is not to define the individual but to express and sustain the communal.[1]

For me, art making has continually helped me know that I am not alone in this life, that I am a part of something much larger, more beautiful, and infinitely more wonderful than my existence as a separate entity. However personally lonely we may feel on occasion, this collective creative source is available all the time.

It always impresses me that when speech and customs form a barrier with others, if I take out pencils and paper, paintbrushes and paint, or a handful of clay, communication and connectedness spontaneously emerge as if a universal language were being spoken. Many years ago I was sent by the Kennedy Center for the Arts to China to teach art therapy to educators and psychologists in Beijing. On the first day I faced a hundred and fifty adults without an interpreter and knew no Chinese, and my students knew very little English. I brought paper, oil pastels, paint, and brushes from home, thinking that there might be very few places to obtain art supplies there. Without words, I demonstrated to the class some simple art techniques, persuading them with my own enthusiasm to join me in creating. The audience spontaneously jumped from their seats, formed groups, and began painting murals on large white paper I provided. At the end of the session, each group stood by its painting, spoke animatedly about the images, and encouraged me to photograph them standing by their creations. Art making is a form of knowing that we all can tap because the act of art making joins us to a creative source that is shared by everyone.

ENTERING THE KARASS

In the novel *Cat's Cradle*, Kurt Vonnegut describes a world where people come together for a common purpose and through an organizational unit he calls a karass. It is basically a group of individuals, from two to several hundred, who are united through a shared goal, sometimes never meeting the others who are invested in that goal. But they are all held in relationship because they all share a similar reason for being in the world.

In recent years, there is a growing movement to redefine the mission of art, transforming it from its position in Western culture as a commodity to a sacred and communal activity. Reminiscent of Vonnegut's notion of the karass, this way of thinking has emerged simultaneously in the art world, psychotherapy, and medicine. Many artists, therapists, and others are seeking ways to use the collective wisdom of art and imagination, envisioning ways that it can become a healing practice for communities of people as well as the world. In contrast to placing art on walls, in museums, or for sale in galleries, there is a quest for ways to use the creative source on behalf of neighborhoods, institutions, and the planet. Art is being used to connect and transform communities through exhibitions of healing art, sacred installations, and art making in communal settings. The future of the soul's palette may indeed be its evolution beyond individualism toward a more inclusive, expansive, and global purpose.

For several decades, many like-minded individuals held a vision for art as a form of therapy, the kernel of the idea that was eventually to become art therapy. Like many other artists, I thought I surely was the first person to recognize art's powers to heal and make whole. I didn't know that I was actually part of a karass that had been forming for a long time. In the late 1970s, I was both shocked and pleasantly surprised to discover that so many others were dedicated to this concept and there were people who called themselves art therapists. I immediately felt held in relationship to people I met or read about in books and journals, people who were on the same path as I was. Chances are that if the ideas in this book resonate with you, you also are part of the karass of art as a healing and transformational practice.

THE ENERGY OF SYNERGY

Making art within a group arouses special energy that extends the dimensions of the creative process. There is a synergistic effect between the space where communal art making takes place and the people within it that is vital and interactive. Shaun McNiff refers to this as a "creative ecology of forces."[2] While the process and the end result of art making are central to its transformative quality, how art makers come together to create emanates its own unique vitality and influence.

If you take a studio art course or simply gather with a few friends or family to make art, you will naturally experience the synergy of being in a creative community. When I make art alongside others, I find myself having a whole new set of experiences, inspirations, and awakenings that don't occur when I am alone in my studio. Sometimes I am an observer, admiring what others are making and taking mental notes about content, style, use of materials, and techniques.

Other times the rhythm of the group seems to overtake me, slowing down my breathing or energizing my creative flow, encouraging me to join the group's tempo and personality. Once in a while I have to learn patience as other art makers lean over my shoulder, interject a comment, or disturb my thinking at what I believe is a critical moment in my creative process. Those instances teach me to become part of a more natural pace of life, one that isn't dependent on deadlines, ego, or outcome but is fluid and flexible to the needs of other people and the environment. Then there are days when I simply enjoy being in a group making art for the fun of it, chatting over a cup of tea, savoring the smell of paint, and watching the visual drama of others at work.

I also rediscover how creating within a group awakens energy in other parts of my life. Experiencing how I fit into a larger context always helps me to see and expand beyond myself. There are individuals with whom I can share joys and discoveries and opportunities to listen to others' stories and for them to be present to mine. This experience inevitably changes my awareness of myself and others, deepening my empathy and regard for each and every human being with whom I come in contact.

Sometimes what we are looking for in both life and artistic expression is more accessible when we do it together. When we make art in the same space, the synergy of the experience nourishes and teaches us in ways we may not find by going it alone.

FINDING A WAY TO CREATE COMMUNITY

Imagine the following:

- A group of breast cancer survivors gathers at a wellness center to paint healing mandalas that will be displayed at the oncology clinic at their local hospital.
- Members of a healing artist's network create a website to display sacred art as a prayer for their communities and the earth.
- A class of fourth-graders draws brightly colored pictures of rainbows and hearts to send to schoolchildren of war-torn Kosovo.

- An artist creates a series of crosses on a hillside in Colorado, and high school students and their families write prayers and create pictures to attach to them, commemorating those who have died in a school shooting.

- Individuals at an art therapy retreat make a labyrinth from stones and found objects and place images for global peace within the center.

- Artists create a sculpture for a pediatric cancer unit and read poems aloud to patients for a month with the intention of healing patients, families, hospital staff, the community, and the earth.

These are just a few of the infinite ways that the creative source, the soul's palette, is being used in communities to heal and transform. These communities exist all around us to join and experience. We can participate in a weekly art studio group with others; we may join an arts medicine program at a hospital outpatient clinic; we may add to the painting of an urban mural on a wall in an inner city; or we might share our drawings on a website so that others can enjoy the images we have made. The AIDS Memorial Quilt is a wonderful and well-known example of a gathering of souls to make art on behalf of others. Sponsored by the Names Project, it has brought millions of people together, both creators and observers, to memorialize the lives of those who have died from AIDS. Other programs in schools, neighborhoods, institutions, prisons, hospitals, homeless shelters, and galleries are less dramatic but bring the same possibility for sharing artistic expression in expansive and powerful ways.

If you envision using your creative source on behalf of others, consider what that image for community art making would be. For more than a decade I have been involved in offering "creativity and wellness groups" to those with cancer or other medical illnesses. Rather than designing a group based on the word *therapy,* my intention was to create a community whose central purpose is commitment to artistic expression as a wellness practice. I hoped that I could facilitate a sense of empowerment and participation in one's own health through using one's creative source as opposed to the traditional medical model that emphasizes a passive role in one's treatment.

As it turned out, the idea was more successful that I could have imagined. Not only did group members, most of whom initially identified themselves as non-artists, like the idea of art as a complement to their health maintenance, they felt validated by a community where a sense of wellness rather than illness was supported. I learned to be less a facilitator in these groups and more of a cocreator, someone who reflected and supported the vision that participants expressed for the group's direction. By taking that role, I continue to learn from these groups the wonders of how art making transforms and ultimately heals.

Try forming your own creativity and wellness group with a small number of friends or colleagues. You can use the activities and practices in this book as an inspiration or simply get together to make art in your own way. The following suggestions may help guide the formation of your group.

Be bold—just get started. Invite friends, family, or colleagues to participate and trust that you will learn what you need to know as the group evolves.

Consider the space. Remember, spaces are what you make of them, and almost any space can be transformed into one for art making. Revisit the suggestions in chapter 4 about designing and creating a studio. You need a space to meet in that allows group members to feel safe, comfortable, and inspired to make art.

Choose a facilitator. While some groups don't need a leader, new ones do need someone to serve as the facilitator to support the process as it initially unfolds. A facilitator is not there to take charge or give directions but is a kind of "holder of the space": by being present to what is taking place, he or she establishes a sense of containment for the group, an important energetic force in communal art making.

You may choose someone to facilitate for a number of weeks or months, or each group member may want to take a turn facilitating the group's meetings in order to share the responsibility. Whoever does the facilitating, it is important to model a presence that supports authentic art expression and heartful acceptance of the creative process as a wellness practice.

Clarify goals and objectives. The path of the group is always open to revision, but in the beginning it is important to clarify how members envision the group's goals and direction. Decide on a format and rules, such as arriving on time, keeping silence during art making, sharing and discussion for the last half hour, confidentiality issues, and whether or not guests are allowed. Determine as a group how often you want to meet and whether the group should be limited to a particular number of days or weeks. Allow members to periodically reevaluate what they think of the group and what new directions they would like to see it take.

Make safety central. In psychotherapy, therapists talk about safety in terms of confidentiality and of creating a place where people can freely express themselves. In art making, a safe space for creative expression encourages free and authentic expression that will be seen by everyone in the group. Spend some time as a group considering and sharing how the group defines safety: for example, no comments about another's artwork unless asked, what is confidential and what is not, sensitivity to each other's needs and process. Be sure to have the facilitator or group periodically evaluate whether the art-making community feels relaxed, comfortable, and open.

Use the power of intention. It is important for group members to create a clear intention for the space, the experience, and the participants. Each person may wish to make an intention for his or her creative work, and the group may wish to express its collective vision for gathering to make art together.

Enhance a sense of community. Consider ways that a sense of community can be enhanced within the group. Rituals can help to build connectedness among members; perhaps each group starts with some playful movement or yoga stretches or a short meditation to allow everyone to become focused. There may be a time when everyone comes together to share a cup of tea and talk about their art, or the group may end with a visualization that suits the collective intention of the participants.

WITNESSING WITH HEART AND MIND

Art making in a group naturally leads to the witnessing of the creative source in others. Witnessing others' images is not at all like the traditional art school "critique," where criticism, analysis, judgment, and opinion prevail. It is more like mindfulness meditation, where one learns to find awareness and nonjudgment without getting caught in thoughts, feelings, and sensations. It is an experience of watching, being with, and listening without attachment or evaluation. In becoming a mindful witness to the stories and images of others, I have been given the opportunity to learn more about the joy as well as the suffering of others. In being present to another's creative source in this way, my own soul has been renewed in directions and dimensions beyond the confines of my own art making.

I have become a student of such mindful witnessing through both experience and practice over a long period of time. In one of my first positions as an art therapist, I worked with children who came from violent homes and who were often abused or neglected. In the beginning I was struck by the intense fears and sadness these children brought to the groups. Their drawings and paintings held their frightening experiences as survivors of beatings or memories of seeing a parent assaulted. The impact on me was immediate; as I witnessed their expressions and heard their stories, I wondered how or if I could be of help to them. On many days I was overwhelmed by the sheer terror of their images and narratives to the point of feeling helpless, hopeless, and tearful. It took me a while to understand how I was of help to these children, but eventually I had an important awakening about the simple importance of being fully present to another's pain and suffering without attachment or judgment. While my skills as a therapist taught me how me to intervene, my own creative source helped me to accept what I saw and heard with my heart as well as my head.

Since that time I have spent most of my life being present to the art of those in emotional, physical, and spiritual pain. In seeing the art of others and witnessing the wonder and mystery of the creative spirit to restore, transcend, and transform, I have been humbled to repeatedly learn what it is to be compassionate and in service to those in need. Compassion truly comes from witnessing the pain that others have suffered as well as our own suffering. I believe that witnessing art without judgment helps us to empathize with others and teaches us about our own wounds. Whether images contain pain and suffering or beauty and wonder, an open heart and a state of mindful awareness are sources for understanding another human being and knowing ourselves. When we create and interact with others within the same art-making space, using both heart and mind can help us to feel deeply and respond wisely.

Consider how you respond to images created by others and ways that you can receive others' images with both heart and mind. The following practices may help you to develop compassion and mindfulness toward others.

Keep a journal about your group work. I find that even a short entry in my journal after a group experience helps me to sort out my reactions to others' images and practice heartful and mindful responses. Use the techniques described in chapter 6 as a starting point for writing, or create images in response to the group process. Use your journal as a way to reflect on the group's evolution as well as your own and your progress with practicing nonattachment and nonjudgment.

Revisit don't-think mind. Experience others' creative source with a beginner's innocence, curiosity, and humility. Remember that not-knowing is one of the best ways to fully and freely open ourselves to the experiences of another; it lets us enjoy surprise, appreciate mystery, and learn new things. Don't-think mind helps us to stay clear of judgment and to respond from the heart.

Be present. As explained in chapter 6, simply being present to your experiences and reactions will strengthen the internal witness and will help you practice nonjudgment. In a communal setting, try to stay present to others' stories and images by acknowledging them and receiving them in the moment. One of the wonderful aspects of working in a group is that everyone gets to witness each other. Being fully present to one another helps us to feel connected in that our deepest joys and pains are seen, heard, and held by others. When our images are received by others in this way, we experience the sacred through being accepted as part of a larger whole.

REACHING OUT BEYOND THE SELF

Janis Timm-Bottos—an artist, art therapist, and community activist—has held a vision for the power of art to build and enhance community for many years. In downtown Albuquerque, New Mexico, she was instrumental in establishing Art Street and, later, Off-Center Studio, two art programs that move art beyond the boundaries of the individual and into urban streets and neighborhoods. Her vision has created spaces for people who may have been disenfranchised by society for reasons of low income or disability to become artists in their own right by making art with other like-minded souls. These studios have become communities in and of themselves. They also have spilled out beyond themselves through storefront galleries and other interactive programs, reaching the entire city and inspiring other programs in communities across the United States.

All around us we are seeing the reflection of Timm-Bottos's and other individuals' intentions for art as a transformer of communities become reality. In my community, an old restaurant was transformed into a walk-in art studio for homeless teenagers; a storefront art studio opens its doors daily to people with disabilities who make art for sale. Raw Art Works, mentioned in chapter 1, is a model for how art expression transforms not only individuals but entire communities. There are a growing number of programs emerging with a similar mission to reach the soul of community through the creative source.

Art expression is an intensely personal experience that transforms on an individual level. But when one uses self-expression to move beyond the boundaries of the self, remarkable transformations occur that touch those around us. Try thinking outside of your own studio and into your neighborhood, town, or even the world about how you can use art in transformative ways. If you look around your city, you are likely to find some sort of community-based program through which you can experience art making in a group. There may be a weekend or weeklong workshop or retreat, or a studio offering group art-making possibilities or opportunities to "drop in" and work in an informal setting where others are creating. If you are physically ill, check with your hospital to find out if there is an arts medicine program or an ongoing art group.

If there is nothing where you live that suits you, don't give up. There are many paths to tapping the power of artistic expression to reach the soul of community:

Search the World Wide Web. Type the words *art* and *healing* into a search engine and you will find numerous art-making communities that you can join without leaving your home. Some of these include:

- The Arts and Healing Network, an international resource for those interested in the healing potential of art

- The Survivors Art Foundation, an international organization dedicated to providing ways for those who have been traumatized to exhibit work through an Internet art gallery and outreach programs

- The ArtsAIDS site, an ongoing Internet project where people can create digital works of art to share their experiences, aimed at enabling artists to participate globally

- ARTS Anonymous, a group supporting those who need support in motivating their creative process.

Start your own community art project. When I was an art professor, each year I filled up Chinese restaurant take-out containers with collage materials, natural objects, and trinkets. I gave the boxes not only to my students but also to the office staff and other non-artist colleagues as an inspiration to make art. We scheduled a time a month later to share with each other what we had created. It gave me great pleasure to make a gift of materials to a group of people and then later have the chance to witness what each one had done.

A group of artist friends recently conceived a similar project, sending out "art seed packets" to others around the country. While not everyone ended up making art from the seed packets, everyone who received one talked about getting it and feeling connected to some larger community. Most recipients dedicated some amount of energy to the process, whether actually making something from the materials or commiserating with others who couldn't find time or were not inspired by what they received. The intention was a success in that it created a group consciousness among people who were separated by distance and lacked a regular connection with one another.

Invent ways that you can stimulate the art process in others. Make a gift of collage materials to friends, donate an Art Rx Box to a cancer ward at your local hospital, take some craft materials to an elderly-care facility, or bring paints and paper to a homeless shelter once a month.

Find an art soulmate or two. There is someone out there who is your "art soulmate," a person who can help to inspire your creativity. I have an art soulmate who lives two thousand miles away; we call each other just to chat about our art and find ways to nurture creativity in each other. Our latest project is a small drawing that we mail back and forth, each adding color, lines, or forms until we decide it is finished and it is time to start a new one. Closer to home, I have another friend with whom I meet every month to make art for several hours on an afternoon when we can both play hooky from work. Look around your circle of friends and colleagues and consider who is a possible candidate to be your art soulmate.

Join a global healing practice. The soul of community is not limited to your own backyard; around the world there are opportunities to use the power of art for transformation and well-being. In Bosnia, humanitarian efforts have been mobilized by organizations such as Doctors Without Borders and ArtReach to bring art to children who have been brutalized by the aftermath of war and terror. The simple act of offering crayons and paper has helped child survivors express their fears and the horrors of their experiences. Similarly, the National Artists for Mental Health offers a project called Pillows of Unrest, encouraging the painting of a pillowcase as a canvas as emotional self-expression and as intention for healing and recovery. The goal is to reduce the stigma that society places on mental illness and to call attention to the healing potential of art making.

§

Think of ways that you can step out beyond the boundaries of your studio space and use your creativity as a way to impact the world. You don't necessarily have to travel to some exotic location to use art for global healing. Think of your creative spirit as a gift, and make art with a sacred intention for those in the world who are suffering, or practice your art as a way of extending your spirit to others, whether in your own community or in behalf of people in need. Imagine both modest and grand ways that your creative source can impact others and how art for well-being can reach as many as possible in your neighborhood or town or the planet.

HEALING ART: FRUITS OF THE BODHISATTVA

Every so often I encounter people who, because of illness or trauma, cannot enjoy all that the soul's palette has to offer and may not be able to pick up a pencil to draw or a brush to paint. A few times in my work as an art therapist I have been called on by people to make images for them when medical conditions have debilitated them so profoundly that it is impossible to do even simple tasks. One young man in the final stages of AIDS asked me to bring his collection of collage images from his home to his hospital bedside and instructed me on how to create a series of cards that would be sent to loved ones upon his death. Another, a woman with terminal cancer, wanted me to paint a mandala for her with specific colors, symbols, and images so that she could have it by her bedside while in the hospital as an image of her religious faith.

I have also been the fortunate recipient of art made by others on my behalf. Once, when I was leaving my post as editor of a journal after nine years of service, a group of friends and colleagues decided to create a visual memory book in honor of the passage. They each made a small painting, drawing, or collage to add to the book along with a personal message. Every page was a work of art, and each was made even more special because of the heart and spirit that was involved in its creation.

That book contains the essence of the healing power of art because embedded in each image are acts of tenderness, friendship, and love. Art made with such intention can be a manifestation of the Buddhist principle of *bodhichitta*, the innate heart of awareness that may lead to acts of compassion. The generosity of my friends and colleagues in creating these images extends the reach of creativity beyond its usual function of self-expression or product to one of altruism and the intention of a bodhisattva.

Many artists are seeking a healing mission for their art beyond commodity. Some work in hospitals, making art for people who cannot use their creative source for reasons of disability or pain, or with people who have limited capabilities because of illness or medical treatment. A growing number of artists say that their aim is to create their art selflessly, in the service of a higher power directed to the good of all. These artists reject the idea of art for art's sake and emphasize making their art an accessible, shared experience, one that reflects a deeper connection to spirit and a higher wisdom.

Christiane Corbat is one such artist who collaborates with individuals with cancer or other serious illness to create a work that reflects on that experience. In her words: "Art influences and transforms life. As an artist I became convinced of this first hand during a personal crisis ten years ago. I made plaster casts of my body and transformed them into mythical, dream-like images which embodied the qualities I wished to have as part of my life. This process not only 'healed' me, it gave me a tool with which to change my life. I asked my friends to help by allowing me to make similarly transformative pieces about their battles with life threatening diseases or with their deepest fears."[3] Corbat's work includes art made in collaboration with people with various forms of cancer and other physical and emotional problems. She believes the symbolic image created from this union transforms experiences of pain, suffering, or disfigurement and helps people to feel whole and healed in spirit, regardless of the state of mind or body.

In the tradition of the Tibetan prayer flag, visionary artists Alex Grey and Allison Grey created a performance and installation piece for a public space at a large hospital that exemplifies true healing art. *Mending the Heart Net* consisted of a large heart surrounded by a twenty-foot rope net. Cut-up bandages and pens were offered along with the invitation to patients, visitors, and staff to write a prayer on a bandage for someone who was ill or to express their own heart's desire. The bandages were pinned to the heart net, eventually covering it with prayers and intentions.

The power of the piece was through both the act of intention underlying the work and the content of the images. While the piece was taken down after two weeks, artists from the hospital's arts in medicine program read the prayers out loud for an additional week. The bandages were eventually tied into a long rope, and the artists again read the prayers aloud. As a final ritual, the prayers were buried in the earth in the center of a nearby tree that had been struck by lightning, thus burning out its center. Like the Tibetan prayer flag, the *Heart Net* was an impermanent piece, but the intentions and prayers are enduring even though the images were destroyed.

Some have used the term "healing artist" to describe one who makes art on behalf of another person's well-being. This term, I believe, may

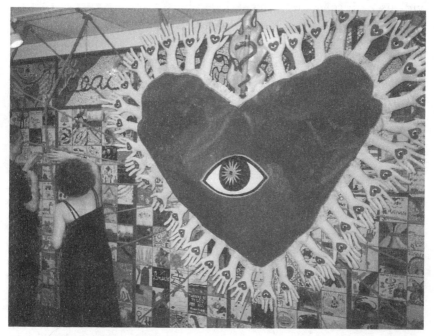

Alex and Allison Grey's *Heart Net*.

be somewhat of a misnomer because it is not actually the artist who does the healing. While the artist contributes understanding and skill in art, what often develops between the artist and the individual is a profound and deep relationship through the intimacy of one person creating for another. The image created as well as the relationship formed embody the possibility for transformation and transcendence, and ultimately an experience of healing for both the art maker and the recipient. In giving of ourselves in this way, we receive the benefits of serving others in a selfless way through our creative source. We create the possibility for well-being and wholeness to emerge within those served as well as ourselves.

How might you commit some of your creative source to helping another person? Try making a special mandala or small sculptural object with specific intentions for a friend or family member in need. A guardian figure, as described in a previous section of this chapter, may be your inspiration to use your imagination on behalf of another person. Your artistic expression can even be a handcrafted item that would comfort another; a quilt or an embroidered pillow can be a special kind of medicine for someone who is ill or experiencing a loss or tragedy. Best of all, committing your creative source in this way will not only touch its recipient, the intention of your action will reverberate in your own life in the process.

ARTFUL INTENTIONS: PAYING IT FORWARD

Several years ago a simple but profound gift was given to me while I was lecturing in Korea. Before I was to begin teaching one morning, the students in my class gave me a bag of one thousand origami paper cranes that they had made. In Korea and Japan, there is a legend that cranes live to be one thousand years old, and the act of folding one thousand paper cranes (called *senbazuru* in Japanese) results in a wish being granted. To give someone one thousand cranes is an auspicious event that holds great power, reverence, and intention. The gift of the origami cranes on that day represented my students' blessings for a wonderful day and good luck in the future. I felt extremely honored to be the recipient of such an act from people whom I did not know. I made a wish in that moment that the magic of the thousand cranes would continue beyond that day in Korea and stay within my life for a long, long time.

The students' generosity in giving me this gift and its intention has grown in depth and unforeseen dimensions for many years. Near the front door of our home a small basket of those paper cranes sits as a daily reminder of a memorable trip and a journey that permanently changed my life. But the miracle of the class's gesture has had an even greater impact than I could have originally imagined. I always keep a handful of those cranes in my handbag and luggage, leaving some with students, friends, or colleagues; at the bedsides of sick children or adults; with counselors or teachers whose schools were sites of shootings or violence; and with others whom I meet in my travels. Every time I pass on a paper crane, I tell a little bit about the group of people I met in Korea and their kindness, and ask the recipients of the cranes to make their own special wish for themselves or someone they love. Those cranes are in the hands of hundreds of other people now throughout the United States, Europe, and Australia. The image and its intention have been passed on, and with each passing, a story of generosity is told and retold and new wishes are made and hopefully fulfilled.

It would be indeed revolutionary if each of us could offer one small act of art to another person. The origami cranes I received are a good example of an artful intention, a single act that eventually "pays it forward" in ways that often cannot be predicted or planned. Paying it forward simply means that if a kindness comes to you, you pass it on to others, without any thought of getting something back in return. One simple act of creative intention can lead to numerous others, like expanding circles in a lake when you cast a stone into the water. When we let our images reach beyond self-expression to symbolic intentions, we create art that cares not only for ourselves but also for the souls of others, even those we do not or may never know. It is a far-reaching act that can extend beyond ourselves and touch the lives of great numbers of people in profound and meaningful ways. It is a practice that we all can use to create connection and to further the potential of the soul's palette not only to transform a community but also to heal and make whole our world.

IMAGES ARE MIRACLES

In bringing the artistic wisdom you have discovered within yourself into a larger community, you reach those deepest parts of yourself through sharing and celebrating this wisdom with others. You awaken creative energy not only within yourself but in those around you. This is a powerful act of intention that extends and deepens your creative source and its powers beyond the self.

Every day we all have the possibility to tap the soul's palette, individually and within community, as a wellness practice for ourselves and others. Artistic expression and imagination are always available to bring well-being to the bodymind, psyche, and spirit and to connect us to that which is sacred, transcendent, and transformative. While there is no question that our creative source enhances wellness, images and the process of image making and imagination are truly miracles. We do not know all there is to know about why artistic creativity heals and makes us whole. Each time we sit in our studio to draw, at an easel to paint, or at a work table to touch clay with the intention of bringing our vision into form, we engage in a mystery that contains our own power to repair, renew, replenish, and restore. It is a miracle in that it takes us beyond ourselves while at the same time bringing us back to ourselves. And each time we engage this mystery, we experience a universal energy that flows through each of us and sets us on a common path, a creative journey, that will inevitably lead us home.

Notes

Chapter 2. Creativity as a Healing Force

1. Cathy A. Malchiodi, "Using Drawing as Intervention with Traumatized Children and Adults," *Trauma and Loss: Research and Intervention*
   1, no. 1 (2001), pp. 21–28.

Chapter 3. Embracing Your Creative Birthright

1. See interview with Satish Kumar in Suzi Gablik, *Conversations before
   the End of Time* (London: Thames & Hudson, 1997), p. 137.
2. For this story and more information on Howard Ikemoto, see the
   following websites: www.brainyquote.com/quotes/authors and
   www.metroactive.com/papers/cruz/11.15.00/ikemoto1-0046.html.

Chapter 5. Visual Symbols as Messengers, Guides, and Friends

1. Henry David Thoreau, *Walden* (Princeton, N.J.: Princeton University
   Press, 1971), p. 323.

Chapter 6. Letting Your Images Tell Their Stories

1. Paolo Knill, Helen Barba, and Margo Fuchs, *Minstrels of the Soul:
   Intermodal Expressive Therapies* (Toronto: Palmerston Press, 1995),
   p. 33.

2. Coleman Barks, *The Essential Rumi* (San Francisco: HarperSanFrancisco, 1997), p. 40.

Chapter 7. Images as a Path to Physical Well-Being

1. See Marc Ian Barasch, *Healing Dreams: Exploring Dreams That Can Transform Your Life* (New York: Riverhead, 2000), p. 73.
2. In Ernest Rossi and David Cheek, *Mind-Body Therapy* (New York: Norton, 1988), pp. 375–76.

Chapter 8. Art as Reparation and Restoration

1. C. G. Jung, *Memories, Dreams, Reflections* (New York: Pantheon, 1961), p. 21.
2. See Roger Ulrich, "View through a Window May Influence Recovery from Surgery," *Scientific American* 224 (1984), pp. 420–21, and Roger Ulrich, "Effects of Healthcare Interior Design on Wellness: Theory and Recent Scientific Research," in *Innovations in Healthcare Design,* Sarah Marberry, ed. (New York: Van Nostrand Reinhold, 1995), pp. 88–104.
3. Rainer Maria Rilke, *Letters to a Young Poet* (New York, Random House, 2001), p. 43.

Chapter 9. Nurturing the Sacred

1. *Silent Teachings of Meher Baba: Discourses and Conversations* (East Windsor, N.J.: Beloved Books, 2001), p. 118.
2. Khenpo Konchog Gyaltshen Rinpoche, "The Power of Windhorse," at website: www.sunray.org/Buddhist/Windhorse/windhorse.html.
3. Pat B. Allen, "Intention and Creativity: Art as a Spiritual Practice," in *The Soul of Creativity,* Toni Pearce Myers (Novato, Calif.: New World Library, 1999), p. 172.

Chapter 10. Sharing the Artist Within

1. See interview with Satish Kumar in Gablik, *Conversations before the End of Time.*
2. Shaun McNiff, "Keeping the Studio," *Art Therapy: Journal of the American Art Therapy Association* 12, no. 3 (1995), pp. 179–83.
3. From Christiane Corbat's website: www.artheals.org/artists/Corbat_Christiane_34.

Bibliography

Achterberg, Jeanne, and Frank Lawlis. 1984. *Imagery and Disease*. Champaign, Ill.: Institute for Personality and Ability Testing.

Allen, Pat B. 1995. *Art Is a Way of Knowing*. Boston: Shambhala Publications.

Arrien, Angeles. 1992. *Signs of Life*. Sonoma, Calif.: Arcus.

Artress, Lauren. 1995. *Walking a Sacred Path: Rediscovering the Labyrinth as a Spiritual Tool*. New York: Riverhead.

Bach, Susan. 1990. *Life Paints Its Own Span*. Zurich: Daimon.

Barasch, Marc Ian. 2000. *Healing Dreams: Exploring Dreams That Can Transform Your Life*. New York: Riverhead.

Campbell, Don. 1997. *The Mozart Effect*. New York: Avon.

Cane, Florence. 1951. *The Artist in Each of Us*. New York: Pantheon.

Cappachione, Lucia. 1988. *The Power of Your Other Hand*. North Hollywood: Newcastle.

Chödrön, Pema. 1998. *Noble Heart*. Boulder: Sounds True. Audio tape.

Chopra, Deepak. 1990. *Quantum Healing: Exploring the Frontiers of Mind–Body Medicine*. New York: Bantam.

Csikszentmihalyi, Mihalyi. 1990. *Flow: The Psychology of Optimal Experience*. New York: Harper & Row.

Dalai Lama. 2001. *An Open Heart: Practicing Compassion in Everyday Life*. New York: Little, Brown & Co.

Dissanayake, Ellen. 1989. *What Is Art For?* Seattle: University of Washington Press.

Dossey, Larry. 1993. *Healing Words: The Power of Prayer and the Practice of Medicine*. New York: HarperCollins.

Dutlinger, Anne. 2000. *Art, Music, and Education as Strategies for Survival*. New York: Herodias.

Erickson, Milton. 2000. *The Letters of Milton Erickson*. Phoenix: Zeig, Tucker & Co.

Fontana, David. 1993. *The Secret Language of Symbols*. San Francisco: Chronicle Books.

Fox, Matthew. 2000. *Original Blessing: A Primer in Creating Spirituality Presented in Four Paths, Twenty-six Themes, and Two Questions*. New York: Putnam.

Gablik, Suzi. 1991. *The Reenchantment of Art*. London: Thames & Hudson.

———. 1997. *Conversations before the End of Time*. London: Thames & Hudson.

Garfield, Patricia. 1991. *The Healing Power of Dreams*. New York: Fireside.

Graham-Pole, John. 2000. *Illness and the Art of Creative Self-Expression*. Oakland, Calif.: New Harbinger.

Grey, Alex. 1998. *The Mission of Art*. Boston: Shambhala Publications.

Grof, Stanislav. 1993. *The Holotropic Mind*. New York: HarperCollins.

Hillman, James. 1991. *A Blue Fire: Selected Writings*. New York: Harper-Perennial.

———. 1979. *The Dream and the Underworld*. New York: Harper & Row.

Jung, C. G. 1959. *Mandala Symbolism*. Princeton, N.J.: Princeton University Press.

———. 1961. *Memories, Dreams, Reflections*. New York: Pantheon.

Kellogg, Joan. 1991. *Mandala: Path of Beauty*. Lightfoot, Va.: MARI.

Knill, Paolo; Helen Barba; and Margo Fuchs. 1995. *Minstrels of the Soul: Intermodal Expressive Therapy*. Toronto: Palmiston Press.

Koff-Chapin, Deborah. 1999. *Drawing Out Your Soul: The Touch Drawing Handbook*. Langley, Wash.: Center for Touch Drawing.

Kornfield, Jack. 1993. *A Path with Heart*. New York: Bantam Doubleday Dell.

Lerner, Michael. 1996. *Choices in Healing*. Cambridge: MIT Press.

London, Peter. 1989. *No More Secondhand Art: Awakening the Artist Within*. Boston: Shambhala Publications.

McNiff, Shaun. 1992. *Art as Medicine: Creating a Therapy of the Imagination*. Boston: Shambhala Publications.

———. 1998. *Trust the Process*. Boston: Shambhala Publications.

Moore, Thomas. 1994. *Care of the Soul*. New York: HarperPerennial.

Myers, Toni Pearce 1999. *The Soul of Creativity: Insights into the Creative Process*. Novato, Calif.: New World Library.

Nachmanovich, Stephen. 1990. *Free Play: Improvisation in Life and Art*. New York: G. P. Putnam & Sons.

Naumburg, Margaret. 1966. *Dynamically Oriented Art Therapy*. New York: Grune & Stratton.

Pennebaker, James. 1997. *Opening Up: The Healing Power of Confiding in Others*. New York: Guilford.

Rico, Gabriele. 1993. *Pain and Possibility: Writing Your Way through Personal Crisis*. Los Angeles: Tarcher.

Sacks, Oliver. 1973. *Awakenings*. New York: Doubleday.

Schulz, Mona Lisa. 1999. *Awakening Intuition:* New York: Three Rivers Press.

Siegel, Bernie. 1986. *Love, Medicine, and Miracles*. New York: Harper.

Timm-Bottos, Janis. 1995. "ArtStreet: Joining Community through Art." *Art Therapy: Journal of the American Art Therapy Association* 12, no. 3.

Van de Castle, Robert L. 1994. *Our Dreaming Mind*. New York: Ballantine.

Virshup, Evelyn. 1979. *Right Brain People in a Left Brain World*. Los Angeles: Art Therapy West.

Vonnegut, Kurt. 1998. *Cat's Cradle*. New York: Delta.

Walker, Barbara. 1983. *Women's Encyclopedia of Myths and Secrets*. San Francisco: HarperSanFrancisco.

———. 1988. *Women's Dictionary of Symbols and Sacred Objects*. San Francisco: HarperSanFrancisco.

Weil, Andrew. 1998. *Eight Weeks to Optimal Health*. New York: Fawcett.

West, Melissa Gayle. 2000. *Exploring the Labyrinth*. New York: Broadway.

Winnicott, Donald. 1971. *Therapeutic Consultations in Child Psychiatry*. New York: Basic Books.

Zukav, Gary. 1990. *The Seat of the Soul*. New York: Fireside.

Resources

Art Supplies

If stores in your area do not carry the materials suggested in this book, try the following art suppliers, which have free catalogues and offer mail-order services:

Daniel Smith
4159 First Avenue South
P.O. Box 84268
Seattle, WA 98124-5568
Phone: (800) 426-7923
Website: www.danielsmith.com

Sax Arts & Crafts
2405 South Calhoun Road
New Berlin, WI 53151
Phone: (800) 558-6696
Website: www.saxarts.com

Music

Music for art making is a personal preference. I usually like music without lyrics during art making because I find it less distracting, and it provides a focus without forcing me to pay attention to it rather than my creative process. Whatever you select should create an uplifting and inspiring mood, so you may have to experiment with a few different kinds of music before you find what works for you. For relaxation during the art process, try music with a rhythm that does not exceed the speed of a relaxed heartbeat (about sixty to seventy beats per minute). There are also a variety of drumming tapes, including shamanic, which some people find enjoyable while engaged in art making. The following are some of my favorite recordings:

Canyon Trilogy by R. Carlos Nakai

Chakra Suite and *Higher Ground* by Steven Halpern

Drums of Passion: The Beat by Babatunde Olatunji

Planet Drum and *Spirit into Sound* by Mickey Hart

Ritual and *Bones* by Gabrielle Roth & the Mirrors

Silk Road Suite and *Mandala* by Kitaro

Narada offers a variety of instrumental music that includes both relaxing and stimulating collections.

Narada
4650 N. Port Washington Road
Milwaukee, WI 53212
Phone: (414) 961-8350
Fax: (414) 961-8351
E-mail: friends@narada.com

Ladyslipper has a wonderful catalog of a variety of music, including instrumental, drumming, and ethnic pieces.

Ladyslipper
P.O. Box 3124-R
Durham, NC 27715
Phone: (919) 383-8773
Fax: (919) 383-3525
Toll-free orders: (800) 634-6044
Email: info@ladyslipper.org

Touch Drawing

Deborah Koff-Chapin, Director
The Center for Touch Drawing
P.O. Box 1089
Langley, WA 98260
Toll-free orders: (800) 989-6334
Fax: (360) 221-5931
E-mail: center@touchdrawing.com
Website: www.touchdrawing.com

Labyrinths

To locate a labyrinth in your area, contact the following organizations.

The Labyrinth Project of Alabama and Southeast
204 Oak Road
Birmingham, AL 35216-1410
Phone: (205) 979-1744
E-mail: AnetRey@aol.com
Website: www.sacredlabyrinth.com/annette

The Labyrinth Society
P.O. Box 144
New Canaan, CT 06840
Phone: (877) 446-4520
E-mail: info@labyrinthsociety.org
Website: www.labyrinthsociety.org

Veriditas, the World-Wide Labyrinth Project
1100 California Street
San Francisco, CA 94108
Phone: (415) 749-6356
E-mail: veriditas@gracecathedral.org
Website: www.gracecathedral.org

Virtual Labyrinths

The following websites offer labyrinths that can be "walked" with your finger directly on the computer screen, or you can download and print images for use as finger labyrinths.

Cretan labyrinths:
Website: www.geocities.com/Yosemite/6182/labig1.html
Website: www.whisperinggrove.com/virtual.htm

Chartres labyrinth:
Website: http://stonecircledesign.com/dsc_vrt_chartres.html

Arts and Healing, Art Therapy, and Expressive Arts Therapies

The American Art Therapy Association (AATA) provides information on art therapy and finding an art therapist in your community.

American Art Therapy Association
1202 Allanson Road
Mundelein, IL 60060-3808
Phone: (888) 290-0878 or (847) 949-6064
Fax: (847) 566-4580
E-mail: info@arttherapy.org
Website: www.arttherapy.org

The Society for the Arts in Healthcare (SAH) provides information on arts programs in hospitals across the United States.

Society for the Arts in Healthcare (main office)
1632 U Street N.W.
Washington, DC 20009
Telephone: (202) 244-8088
Fax: (202) 244-1312
E-mail: mail@TheSAH.org
Website: www.societyartshealthcare.org

The Survivors Art Foundation is dedicated to encouraging healing through the arts and is committed to empowering trauma survivors with effective expressive outlets via an Internet art gallery, outreach programs, national exhibitions, publications, and development of employment skills.

Survivors Art Foundation
P.O. Box 383
Westhampton, NY 11977
E-mail: safe@survivorsartfoundation.org
Website: www.survivorsartfoundation.org

ARTS (Artists Recovering through the Twelve Steps) Anonymous is a fellowship of artists who share their experience, strength, and hope with each other that they may recover from their common problem and help others to surrender to their creativity. There are no dues or fees for ARTS membership; they are self-supporting through their own contributions.

ARTS Anonymous
P.O. Box 230175
New York, NY 10023
Phone: (212) 873-7075
Website: www.pagehost.com/arts

RAWART Works (RAW) is a nonprofit art therapy organization, was founded in 1988, committed to taking art into the streets, public housing, youth incarceration facilities, clinics, soup kitchens, schools, and homes.

RAWART Works
37 Central Square
Lynn, MA 01901
Phone: (781) 593-5515
E-mail: rawartworks@aol.com
Website: www.rawart.org

The International Arts-Medicine Association (IAMA) is an organization dedicated to promoting the use of all the arts as a complement to traditional medical treatment.

International Arts-Medicine Association
714 Old Lancaster Road
Bryn Mawr, PA 19010
Phone: (610) 525-3784
Fax: (610) 525-3250

The Institute of Noetic Sciences supports programs that use art as a healing or transformational tool.

Noetic Arts Program
Institute of Noetic Sciences
101 San Antonio Road
Petaluma, CA 94952
Phone: (707) 775-3500
Fax: (707) 781-7420
E-mail: webmaster@noetic.org

The International Expressive Arts Therapies Association (IEATA) provides information on all the expressive arts therapies—art, music, dance/movement, drama, and poetry—and can direct you to expressive arts therapists in your community and throughout the world.

International Expressive Arts Therapies Association
P.O. Box 320399
San Francisco, CA 94132-0399
Phone: (415) 522-8959
Website: www.ieata.org

The Arts and Healing Network has an extensive website dedicated to promoting artists and arts programs engaged in healing and transformational practices. It is worth visiting just to see the large, inspirational collection of art on exhibit by artists who are part of this network. The website also provides information and contact information on healing arts programs throughout the United States.

Arts & Healing Network
Website: www.artheals.org